BEHAVIORAL TREATMENT
FOR PERSISTENT INSOMNIA

Pergamon Titles of Related Interest

Becker/Heimberg/Bellack SOCIAL SKILLS TREATMENT FOR
DEPRESSION

Gotlib TREATMENT OF DEPRESSION:
An Interpersonal Systems Approach

Hersen/Kazdin/Bellack THE CLINICAL PSYCHOLOGY
HANDBOOK

Last/Hersen HANDBOOK OF ANXIETY DISORDERS

Meichenbaum STRESS INOCULATION TRAINING

Related Journals

(Free sample copies available upon request)

JOURNAL OF ANXIETY DISORDERS
CLINICAL PSYCHOLOGY REVIEW

PSYCHOLOGY PRACTITIONER GUIDEBOOKS
EDITORS

Arnold P. Goldstein, Syracuse University
Leonard Krasner, Stanford University and SUNY at Stony Brook
Sol L. Garfield, Washington University in St. Louis

BEHAVIORAL TREATMENT FOR PERSISTENT INSOMNIA

PATRICIA LACKS
Washington University in St. Louis

PERGAMON PRESS
New York • Oxford • Beijing • Frankfurt
São Paulo • Sydney • Tokyo • Toronto

U.S.A	Pergamon Press, Maxwell House, Fairview Park, Elmsford, New York 10523, U.S.A.
U.K.	Pergamon Press, Headington Hill Hall, Oxford OX3 0BW, England
PEOPLE'S REPUBLIC OF CHINA	Pergamon Press, Room 4037, Qianmen Hotel, Beijing, People's Republic of China
FEDERAL REPUBLIC OF GERMANY	Pergamon Press, Hammerweg 6, D-6242 Kronberg, Federal Republic of Germany
BRAZIL	Pergamon Editora, Rua Eça de Queiros, 346, CEP 04011, Paraiso, São Paulo, Brazil
AUSTRALIA	Pergamon Press Australia, P.O. Box 544, Potts Point, N.S.W. 2011, Australia
JAPAN	Pergamon Press, 8th Floor, Matsuoka Central Building, 1-7-1 Nishishinjuku, Shinjuku-ku, Tokyo 160, Japan
CANADA	Pergamon Press Canada, Suite No. 271 253 College Street, Toronto, Ontario, Canada M5T 1R5

Copyright © 1987 Pergamon Books Inc.

First edition 1987

Library of Congress Cataloging in Publication Data
Lacks, Patricia.
Behavioral treatment for persistent insomnia.
(Psychology practitioner guidebooks)
Bibliography: p.
Includes indexes.
1. Insomnia—Treatment.   2. Behavior therapy.
I. Title.   II. Series.   [DNLM: 1. Behavior Therapy.
2. Insomnia—therapy. WM 188 L141b]
RC548.L33   1987   616.8'49   87–6986

British Library Cataloguing in Publication Data
Lacks, Patricia
Behavioral treatment for persistent
insomnia.—(Psychology practitioner
guidebooks).
1. Insomnia—Treatment   2. Behavior therapy
I. Title   II. Series
616.8'49   RC548
ISBN 0–08–034318–X Hardcover
ISBN 0–08–034317–1 Flexicover

Reproduced, printed and bound in Great Britain by
Hazell Watson & Viney Limited,
Member of the BPCC Group,
Aylesbury, Bucks

This book is for
my son Jeffrey and my daughter Amy

Contents

List of Tables

Preface

This book represents the culmination of 6 years of research that began in 1980. At that time my colleague Amy Bertelson and I joined together in collaboration on a program of research to understand the causes and effective interventions for persistent insomnia. Her background in sleep pathology and sleep laboratory assessment complemented my own interests in behavioral medicine and health promotion. Since then, we have conducted seven treatment outcome studies as well as a number of other nontreatment studies. When we began this program of investigation there was no complete research protocol or treatment manual to follow. Bits and pieces were available from previous studies and I am grateful to the researchers who shared the fruits of their labors so willingly. A great deal of our effort, however, has gone into designing and repeatedly revising the methods and instruments that we have used to recruit, screen, diagnose, treat, assess, and follow up the participants who served as our subjects. I have attempted in this book to present as fully as space would allow the results of our efforts. In particular, we devoted a great deal of time to developing a detailed treatment manual for our therapists. By relying on this manual, we were able to train relatively inexperienced graduate student therapists quickly and to standardize our therapeutic procedures. Chapters 6, 7, and 8 present this treatment manual.

Literally hundreds of individuals contributed to the development of the knowledge presented in this book. By far the largest group of contributors were the subjects themselves—over 400 men and women from the St. Louis area who devoted many hours to the paperwork that allowed us to accomplish our empirical goals. For every hour of service that they received from us, they gave back over an hour to fill out the never-ending forms. In addition to my collaborator Amy Bertelson, two colleagues served major roles as consultants or occasional co-investigators: Martha Storandt who heads the clinical gerontology training program in our department and James Walsh, Director of the Deaconess Hospital Sleep Disorders Center.

Usually a research program of this scope is made possible by a large government grant. Unfortunately, we were in the wrong place at the wrong time as substantial support was not available for this kind of undertaking during these years. However, we did receive a steady supply of small research grants that we were able to stretch to very effective use (BRSG grant numbers S07 RR07054–17 and S07 RR07054–20 awarded by the Biomedical Research Grant Program, Division of Research Resources, National Institute of Health; and National Institute on Aging Training Grant AG00030).

Without copious research funds, this series of investigations would not have been possible if we had not been doing our work at a place like Washington University. We were blessed with a large number of highly competent and motivated graduate and undergraduate students who were eager to trade their efforts for research experience. Some of these students made major and continuing contributions, serving more as colleagues than research assistants. In alphabetical order they are: Mark A. Cook, Teresa White Cook, Ruth Davies, Andrea Jacobs, John Kunkel, Leslie Gans Luchene, Kimberly Powlishta, Saundra Schoicket, Kimberly Sloan, and Jeffrey Sugerman. A group of our clinical psychology graduate students also served as therapists: Lauren Becker, Ruth Davies, Jane Goldmuntz, Linda Kuisk, Michael Kuttner, Daniel Levin, Marguerite Malone, Carla Paganelli, Robin Puder, Angela Rosenberg, and Saundra Schoicket. If it is true that an army travels on its stomach, a research program travels very much as a result of the labors of its research assistants. We had the help of many marvelously talented undergraduate students. Most of them were bound for graduate school and eager to be initiated into the world of research. They made many creative additions to our enterprise. Several of them worked with us for an extended period of time: Daniel Cody, Michaela Kiernan, Rhonda Krivosha, Cynthia Meiners, Susan Orton, and Monique Rotert. The others are: Naomi Arffa, Matthew Eisenberg, Sandra Herrmann, Tina Humm, Ellen Levy, Regina Neumann, Sarah Robinson, Douglas Stewart, Michael Tavill, Erin Wikes, and Wendy Zeppelin.

I also owe appreciation to Jerry Frank and Mary Grace Luke of the Pergamon staff and to copyeditor Jamie Forbes for their skillful and patient editorial assistance. Finally, I would like to thank my husband Paul Gawronik and my children Jeffrey and Amy Lacks who were remarkably understanding and tolerant of my preoccupation and fatigue as I wrote this book. They were very supportive of my efforts and cheerfully took on some of my family responsibilities during this period.

Chapter 1
The Nature of Persistent Insomnia

Sleep is a very important commodity in our society. The common familial morning greeting, "Did you sleep well?" is one indication of the significance we attach to a night of rest. In fact, a large percentage of the population is relatively obsessed with getting a "good night's sleep." We live in a world where too many people lead exceedingly busy, pressure-filled lives. The busier people get, the more concern they have for getting adequate rest in order to fulfill their daytime responsibilities. Because most people have had occasional nights of sleeplessness, they are well acquainted with its debilitating effects upon energy level, work efficiency, and mood.

Occasional nights of sleep loss can evolve into a more chronic pattern of insomnia. The more sleep individuals lose, the more desperate they become to find a remedy. Large numbers turn to sleep medications as the most expedient method of obtaining relief from sleep disturbance. However, long-term use of these drugs brings with it another set of problems and does not provide consistent, restorative sleep. The purpose of this book is to provide the behavior therapist with the necessary information and techniques to be able to offer a nondrug alternative treatment to those who suffer from persistent insomnia.

A detailed treatment manual for the diagnosis and remediation of the complaint of insomnmia comprises over one third of this book. However, even though the procedures are described in considerable detail, they will only be effective if the therapist has sufficient knowledge of sleep and insomnia. Individuals who seek aid for insomnia have many questions about sleep disturbance and related topics. Many poor sleepers also have a worried, obsessive personality style. As a result, they expect the therapist to be an expert and they do not respond well to wavering or hedged statements. Lack of knowledge on the therapist's part will thus result in a crisis of confidence for the

1

participants and make them less willing to engage in the complicated directions that they will be given. The therapist cannot be expected to know everything about this area, but a certain minimum is essential. An excellent overview of the topic is provided by Dement's brief and highly readable 1976 book. A list of this and other recommended readings that will help the therapist to gain the necessary level of understanding is supplied near the end of the book.

In addition to material that the potential insomnia therapist can acquire elsewhere, the first chapters of this book present a detailed introduction to the requisite background information for work in this area. The present chapter covers the definition of insomnia, prevalence of the problem, the typical consequences of persistent sleeplessness, and why treatment with sleep medications is ineffective and sometimes dangerous.

Chapters 2 and 3 present a summary of the current knowledge about sleep processes and sleep disorders. This information will aid the therapist to assess complaints of sleep disturbance and to make an educated judgment as to whether behavioral interventions are the treatment of choice. Some sleep disturbances have an organic basis and can be life-threatening if not given proper medical attention.

Chapter 4 introduces the reader to the most prominent behavioral principles and interventions for alleviation of persistent insomnia. A brief overview of the research findings is also provided, which reveals that stimulus control techniques appear to have the highest efficacy. (A simulus control treatment package constitutes most of the treatment manual that is the focus of this practitioner guidebook.) In chapter 5, the practitioner is guided through the assessment process; 8 measures are included that are specific to this diagnostic activity. Finally, throughout the book a good deal of extra attention is given to the sleep problems of the older adult. There is a strong correlation between sleep disturbance and age; the prevalence of insomnia increases substantially with aging. It is likely that many individuals who request help for insomnia will be older adults.

DEFINITION OF INSOMNIA

Almost all of us have had an occasional sleep-disrupted night before a vacation, paper presentation, or job interview, or because we had too much to drink at a party. Many of us have had brief periods of sleepless nights during periods of stress on the job, the acute period of divorce negotiations, the last trimester of pregnancy, the week after returning from Europe, or during our own illness or that of someone close to us. Some of us have had sleep problems that are regular and persistent for longer periods, say 6 months or even as long as 20 years. Often we can't relate these latter sleep problems to any specific current process although we may be able to identify some precipitating event. All of these types of sleep disruption represent some form of the very heterogeneous set of problems known as insomnia.

Insomnia is not a disease or a diagnostic category in itself; it is a symptom, like fever or chest pain, that requires a careful differential diagnosis. In fact, many sleep experts refer to the *complaint of insomnia*, because the problem is a subjective experience of daytime fatigue, disrupted functioning, or disturbed mood attributed to insufficient sleep at night. However, there is no standard definition of insufficient sleep because the amount of sleep required for a feeling of restedness varies widely among individuals. Each of us has a personal optimum sleep requirement to feel and function at our best. Some require an uninterrupted 10 hours of solid sleep while others lead happy, productive lives with only 3 hours each night. The magic number of 8 hours that is often touted as the "correct" amount of time to sleep is only an average figure collapsed across the population of healthy adults; many of us get less, some may require more.

Available objective indices of sleep may or may not verify an individual's report of curtailed sleep. How to interpret a person's complaint of disturbed sleep in the absence of such objective corroboration is a source of controversy among the researchers and clinicians who specialize in this area. Some investigators would contend that there is no sleep disorder present, while others believe that the objective instrumentation is still too primitive to document all disruptions of sleep.

Insomnia is not only a subjective disorder but a heterogeneous one. For different individuals, the primary symptoms can vary widely in type, intensity, frequency, causative factors, and daytime consequences. Perhaps the most common way of categorizing the complaint of insomnia is according to the time of night when sleep is most disturbed. About 75% of poor sleepers have *sleep onset* insomnia, or trouble getting to sleep at the beginning of the night. Once these people do get to sleep (which may take up to several hours), their sleep during the remainder of the night is not necessarily disrupted. The second most common type of disrupted sleep is *sleep maintenance* insomnia, or sleep that is interrupted in the middle of the night. Sleep maintenance problems can take the forms of waking in the middle of the night accompanied by difficulty returning to sleep, or of waking for many brief intervals. A third type is *early morning awakening*, when the person arouses before the desired time. In addition, poor sleepers may experience poor quality sleep that is too light, restless, and disturbed, or they may have sleep that is inconsistent from night to night and therefore can never be relied on. People who complain of insomnia may have any one of these problems or can suffer from several or the whole set. Their complaint may also shift over time from one to another of these problems.

Another way of categorizing sleep problems is by intensity — as mild, moderate or severe. Duration of the problem is addressed by the categories of transient, persistent, or intermittent. Furthermore, sleep disruption is often classified in terms of its causative factors, such as psychiatric disturbance, medical conditions, or organic sleep pathology.

There is no totally accepted standard definition of insomnia among sleep researchers and clinicians. However, a widely used, multifaceted criterion of insomnia would be:

- Sleep onset latency of more than 30 minutes or
- Awake time during the night totaling more than 30 minutes or
- Less than 6 1/2 total hours of sleep in a night
- Experience of daytime fatigue accompanied by mood and performance decrements
- Symptoms that occur 3 or more nights per week
- Symptom duration of at least several months

Information that will allow the practitioner to make a more thorough diagnosis of insomnia will be presented in chapters 3 and 5.

PREVALENCE OF THE PROBLEM

According to Hauri (1982), each year approximately 10 million Americans will consult their physicians about difficulties with sleep. Of these, about half will be given a prescription for some kind of sleeping medication. Yet these numbers probably represent only a fraction of the people who are troubled about the quality of their sleep. Some estimates of the size of this group are as high as 50 million to 100 million people. In fact, one Gallup poll (1979) found that only 5% of the adult population reported that they *never* had trouble with sleep. That survey also found that 75% reported they sometimes have trouble sleeping and that 20% claimed their sleep was a serious problem.

A number of large-scale surveys have documented the prevalence of insomnia in the United States (e.g., Karacan et al., 1976b). Mellinger, Balter, and Uhlenhuth (1985) report data from a nationally representative sample survey of 3161 noninstitutionalized adults, ages 18 to 79 years. Thirty-five percent indicated that they had some difficulty during the past year with falling asleep or remaining asleep. Half of these reported that the problem bothered them a lot. Of this latter group with serious sleep problems, 36% experienced only difficulty falling asleep, 27% only had trouble staying asleep, and 36% were bothered by both problems. A large-scale survey of representative households in the Los Angeles area (Bixler, A. Kales Soldatos, J. D. Kales & Healey, 1979) also found that 32% of their sample had a current complaint of insomnia and another 10% reported they had experienced this sleep problem in the past. A nationwide survey of over 4000 physicians showed that 18% of patients complained of insomnia (Bixler, J. D. Kales, Scharf, A. Kales & Leo, 1976).

Insomnia is somewhat more frequently reported among women and those of lower educational and socioeconomic status. Sleep disturbance often starts early in life and persists across many years. For 18% of poor sleepers in one survey, the problem began before age 20. The majority of insomniacs (84%) had experienced their problem for more than a year; 40% had suffered from insomnia for over 5 years (Bixler et al., 1979). Among those seeking treatment for poor sleep, the mean duration of the problem is 14 years with ranges up to 30 or 40 years. The most consistent relationship, however, has been one with age. All surveys find that sleeping problems increase with age. For example, Mellinger et al. (1985) found that the prevalence of serious insomnia increased from 14% for those 18 to 34 years old to 25% among the 65-to-79 age group. The pattern of insomnia also changes with age. Younger adults are more likely to complain of difficulty getting to sleep but once asleep they generally sleep through the night. Older adults are more often bothered by lengthy waking periods during the night or by awakening too early in the morning. Much less is known about the incidence of sleep disorders among children and adolescents. One study revealed that 13% of the adolescent population suffers from persistent insomnia and that an additional 38% report occasional bouts of poor sleep (Price, Coates, Thoresen, & Grinstead, 1978).

In summary, surveys of the sleep patterns of American adults substantiate a rather consistent pattern. Insomnia is a widespread and persistent problem. About 18% of adults surveyed report serious current problems with insomnia, while approximately another 18% report mild to moderate current difficulties. Another 10% to 15% report having had problems in the past. More women than men report sleep problems, and sleep complaints increase with age.

CONSEQUENCES OF CHRONIC LACK OF SLEEP

Although insomnia occurs during the night, it has a 24-hour-a-day effect upon the individual's functioning. For many people, the multiple consequences of chronic lack of sleep are much more than just minor annoyances. The ability to work, engage in social activities, and to derive pleasure from their life is seriously compromised by long-term sleep deprivation. What is striking about the effects of persistent insomnia is the broad scope of distress that is reported by the typical sufferer. Having insomnia for any length of time colors all aspects of the person's life and profoundly affects mood, health, interpersonal relations, and work performance. Insomniacs look at the world through gray-colored glasses. Eventually they develop a sense of desperation about their quest for a good night's sleep. Many times their presenting complaints are of the aftereffects of their lack of sleep rather than the insomnia itself.

One of the most prevalent consequences of persistent insomnia is a feeling of low self-esteem or incompetence based on a sense of loss of control over one's life. It is interesting that, despite the large numbers of the population who experience occasional or chronic interference with sleep, many insomniacs feel that their numbers are small and that they are all alone when they are awake in the middle of the night. A large number of insomniacs are embarrassed about their problem and feel that there is some sort of stigma attached to being a poor sleeper. If they do seek treatment for their sleep problems, they are reluctant for anyone else to know about it. Spouses and friends who do not have sleep difficulties have trouble understanding and may urge the insomniac to try harder, to just relax, to do what comes naturally for the good sleeper. Because those who sleep well do so without thinking about it or putting forth any effort, they are hard pressed to come up with any specific or constructive advice. Good sleepers may be somewhat suspicious about someone who cannot sleep easily. They may express the opinion that "it's all in the mind" or that the poor sleeper really gets much more rest than claimed.

The insomnia sufferer does not like the label "insomniac"; perhaps it sounds too much like maniac. To many, having insomnia means that you have some kind of psychological disorder. Dement (1983) reports that in a small study of the patients of 10 family practice physicians, only 4% volunteered that they had a sleep problem, yet in a later interview in which sleep disorders were solicited 30% had a real sleep complaint. Perhaps the insomnia sufferer has learned not to volunteer sleep complaints because of the negative or not too helpful response that such an admission brings. The experience of not being understood only adds to the poor sleeper's feelings of frustration, anxiety, and anger.

There is no reason for a lack of response to a complaint of persistent insomnia. The symptoms are real, extensive, and costly to an individual's life. The complaints are also quite consistent across individuals.

First, there is a feeling of daytime sleepiness. Although the person can maintain an attitude of alertness when necessary, he or she may fall asleep or feel very drowsy during sedentary activities. Insomniacs also feel awful — grouchy, irritable, nonenergetic, and mildly depressed. As a consequence, their interpersonal and marital relations may suffer. Johnson and Spinweber (1983) had Profile of Mood States scores for 278 navy sailors. When subjects were divided into five categories of their subjective estimates of quality of sleep (from *very good* to *very poor*), there was a significant linear relationship between sleep quality and mood on all the scales. Those who described their sleep as poor rated themselves as more tense, depressed, angry, fatigued, and confused, and as having less vigor than those who rated their sleep in more favorable terms. Ratings between the bottom and top sleep quality categories varied by a factor of almost 2 up to 4 times. According to Hauri (1979), "Humans report that almost anything takes greater effort to accomplish after sleep deprivation; they are generally serious, listless, and grim. Spontaneity is missing, and people feel washed out, depleted, without reserves" (p. 254). In research on the effects of sleep curtailment, subjects who were only allowed 4 to 5 hours of sleep per night felt less happy, friendly, and energetic than when allowed their usual amount of rest. These mood changes persisted even after weeks and months of curtailed sleep — the volunteers did not adapt to the lesser amount of rest (Johnson & MacLeod, 1973).

In addition to discomfort and a general sense of malaise from inadequate sleep, individuals with insomnia more frequently report multiple, persistent, and recurrent general health problems. They are hospitalized more often and for longer periods of time than those who do not experience insomnia. They also report that they are more frequently limited in their work by health problems (Bixler et al., 1979). A similar pattern is evident for mental health problems. Poor sleepers are much more likely to report that life is a strain, that they are more nervous and less happy than others, and that they feel the future is hopeless. In fact, insomnia sufferers consistently score higher on measures of depression than good sleepers.

However, Hauri (1979) claims that the dysphoria of the insomniac is not a true depression. Those who have experienced both true depression and the aftereffects of sleep deprivation can tell the difference in the two mood states. The listlessness and depleted feelings of the chronic insomniac are more akin to the feelings described by volunteers in sleep deprivation experiments. One must also consider the chicken/egg issue. Many poor sleepers report that feelings of dysphoria developed *after* they began to experience consistent sleep problems, not before. Over a period of time, as they experienced lowered efficiency and irritable mood, insomniacs developed a sense of frustration and then hopelessness as their multiple attempts to improve their sleep proved futile. These people see the depressive feelings as another consequence of continuing sleep problems rather than as the initial cause. Of course, individuals who do suffer from classical depression are also likely to have sleep complaints, making a differential diagnosis crucial. Treatment for depression with sleep complaints will differ from that employed for sleep complaints accompanied by feelings of depression.

Another area of disrupted functioning for poor sleepers is job performance. While they can manage routine work without too much difficulty, poor sleepers have much more of a problem with those job aspects that are more complicated, take more effort, or require a special level of motivation or ability such as creativity. For example, a clinical psychologist who slept poorly the night before, may not have particular trouble scoring an intelligence test or proofreading a letter, but may find that writing a test report or a manuscript is much more burdensome.

Investigators have emphasized that healthy volunteers can function quite adequately after experimentally induced total sleep deprivation for a few nights. This claim contrasts dramatically with the insomniac's complaint of incapacitation after losing only a few hours sleep. However, for Hauri (1979) the comparison between the two groups is not a fair one. The poor sleeper may have had years of losing several hours of sleep a number of nights per week, depleting any reserves that might be available to cope with fatigue. Poor sleepers have been found to show a greater reaction to experimental sleep deprivation than have sound sleepers. Some researchers (e.g., Carskadon et al., 1976) have suggested that the insomniac's fatigue and performance decrements may be more the consequence of nighttime arousals or the disruption of sleep rather than of the absolute amount of lost sleep.

Volunteers who have been experimentally sleep deprived do perform poorly on tasks of vigilance, reaction time, and simple arithmetic. Fifteen college student insomniacs were given two performance tasks over a 4-week period during which the students filled out daily sleep diaries. Decrements in both morning and afternoon performance were found on the two tasks following a poor night's sleep (Bootzin & Engle-Friedman, 1981). One reason for interference on these types of tasks is that after a certain amount of sleep deprivation, the body starts robbing a few seconds of microsleep, resulting in short lapses of attention. With greater loss of sleep, these lapses increase in number and duration (Hauri, 1979).

Only one study has documented the effects of poor sleep upon job performance. Johnson and Spinweber (1983) studied the relationship of perceived quality of sleep to performance in the navy for 1827 sailors over a period of 6 years. Of these, 1530 (84%) described themselves as good sleepers and 297 (16%) as poor sleepers. Mean subjective sleep onset latency for the good sleepers was less than 20 minutes, whereas for the poor sleepers it averaged over 60 minutes. On workdays, most of the good sleepers reported sleeping 7 to 8 hours per night, whereas the poor sleepers averaged 5 to 7 hours. The career history in the navy was monitored for these individuals for 2 to 4 years. At enlistment, there were no differences between the good and poor sleepers on age, education, or intelligence test scores. However, on measures of career performance, as time passed, the poor sleepers were the less effective sailors. On all the signs of career advancement, poor sleepers performed significantly less well than good sleepers. They received fewer promotions and so remained at lower pay grades; they were less frequently recommended for reenlistment; and they had higher rates of attrition. They were not, however, greater disciplinary problems.

In summary, insomnia is a major health problem that increases health risks and reduces the quality of life for a sizable group of people. The effects of poor sleep are experienced across a wide range of areas including emotional distress, physical illness and hospitalization, interpersonal and marital discord, and vocational inefficiency. In addition, family members, friends, and co-workers are indirectly affected by the poor sleeper's problems.

TREATMENT WITH HYPNOTIC AND SEDATING DRUGS

What are the most common treatments for insomnia? Many people turn first to some home remedy like taking a warm bath or drinking warm milk at bedtime, using eye shades or ear plugs, buying a new mattress, listening to relaxing recordings, or counting sheep in bed. Others may try an over-the-counter sleep preparation or even common aspirin. Probably the most dangerous sleep aid used by large numbers of those seeking slumber is alcohol. If no relief is forthcoming, the largest number of insomnia sufferers will then turn to their personal physicians for help. At least half of these individuals will be given some kind of sleep medication.

Sleep medication is any preparation that promotes sleep or that the insomniac believes will promote sleep. Table 1.1 shows some of the large number of compounds that are currently available for this purpose

Table 1.1. Drugs Most Commonly Prescribed as Hypnotic
Medications

Generic Name	Trade Name
Barbiturates	
Amobarbital	Amytal
Butabarbital	Butisol
Pentobarbital	Nembutal
Phenobarbital	Luminal
Secobarbital	Tuinal, Seconal
Benzodiazepines	
Alprazolam	Xanax
Chlordiazepoxide	Librium
Clorazepate	Tranxene
Diazepam	Valium
Flurazepam	Dalmane
Lorazepam	Ativan
Oxazepam	Serax
Temazepam	Restoril
Triazolam	Halcion
Non-Benzodiazepines	
Chloral hydrate	Noctec, Somnos
Ethchlorvynol	Placidyl
Ethinamate	Valmid
Glutethimide	Doriden
Methaqualone	Parest, Quaalude
Methyprylon	Noludar
Antidepressants	
Amitriptyline	Elavil
Doxepin	Sinequan
Trazodone	Desyrel
Tranquilizers	
Meprobamate	Equanil, Miltown
Thioridazine	Mellaril
Other	
Diphenhydramine	Benadryl
L-Tryptophan	Tryptacin

Note. This table was compiled from three sources: Bertelson (1984), Lichstein and Fischer (1985), and *Physician's desk reference* (1986).

including antidepressants and tranquilizers. In a sample of 216 insomniacs treated in our own research program, 35% were using sleep
medications at the time they contacted us for behavior therapy; many
more had used these remedies at some time in the past. Of the current
medication users, 57% were taking benzodiazepines (mostly Dalmane
or Valium), 12% were taking antidepressants, 17% used over-the-
counter preparations, 5% took barbiturates, and 8% used some other

type of medication. Drugs for sleep were being used an average of 3 nights a week with a range of 1 to 7 nights. Our volunteers had been taking these preparations an average of 7 years with a range from several months up to 30 years.

The most common method for treating insomnia is some kind of sleep-inducing medication grouped under the common heading of *hypnotics*. Even though during the past 15 years there has been an overall decline in the number of this kind of prescription written, the use of medications to promote sleep remains widespread. In 1977, physicians gave nearly 26 million prescriptions for hypnotic medications (Institute of Medicine, 1979). Daniel Kripke, a nationally known sleep researcher, estimates current usage at about 40 million yearly prescriptions (Kripke, 1983). These numbers, however, represent an underestimate of the number of people who take hypnotics because many individuals share their sleeping pills with spouses, relatives, friends, and co-workers. In a large-scale national survey of psychotherapeutic drug use in 3161 individuals, Mellinger et al. (1985) found that 2.6% of the general population had used hypnotics during 1979. Kripke (1983) conservatively estimates the financial cost in 1981 of drug treatment for troubled sleep in this country to fall between $500 million and $1 billion.

In addition to drugs given for outpatient treatment, about one fourth of the over 1 million hospitalized patients receive some sleep medication on any given night whether they ask for it or not. There are also special concerns about the large number of older adults who are given hypnotics. Although the elderly make up only 11% of the United States population, it is estimated that they consume 25% to 40% of the nation's prescription drugs with hypnotics making up a good portion of these. Sleeping pills are extensively used in skilled nursing facilities in which at least 35% of the patients receive hypnotics. In a telephone survey regarding insomnia, half of a sample of 100 noninstitutionalized people over age 65 reported using sleep medication "every night" or "frequently" (Kripke, 1983; Kripke, Ancoli-Israel, Mason, & Messin, 1983).

In another study, 74% of those who had used hypnotics in the past year reported that their longest period of regular daily use was less than 14 days, and 64% had used the drugs for fewer than 30 total days during the year. On the other hand, 11% reported using sleep medications regularly for 12 months or longer, and 19% said they had used the drugs for a total of 120 days or more during the year (Mellinger et al., 1985).

Before 1970, most hypnotic prescriptions were for some type of barbiturate. As recently as 1965, enough barbiturates were being sold in this country to make 6 billion doses. Of all the hypnotics, barbiturates have the most serious side-effects, including the development of tolerance and the potential for addiction and for accidental or planned overdose. There are still an average of 1400 annual deaths from barbiturate overdose (Kripke, 1983). With their introduction in 1970, the benzodiazepines have largely supplanted the barbiturates because they are more effective and less dangerous. Two thirds of all prescribed hypnotics are now from the benzodiazepines, mostly flurazepam (Dalmane).

On the face of it, a pill that promotes sleep would seem to be an ideal remedy for insomnia. Pills are inexpensive, convenient, and simple to take. It is true that most of the currently available prescription hypnotics will show an initial ability to improve or lengthen sleep if the appropriate dosage is prescribed. This added sleep is likely, however, to total only 20 to 40 minutes. Unfortunately, sleep medications usually do not continue to work over any appreciable length of time. Tolerance to many hypnotics develops within 2 weeks, thus requiring increased dosage that may lead to addiction and even to accidental death from overdose. The benzodiazepines appear to maintain their effectiveness for the longest amount of time; however, research has established this benefit only for a period of 4 weeks. Over-the-counter preparations generally have antihistamines as their principle ingredient and may make a person drowsy but are not particularly effective in promoting sleep (Hauri, 1982).

Although hypnotics can effect a short-term improvement in sleep, large numbers of poor sleepers are chronic users of these drugs. After the initial improvement, hypnotics may actually cause insomnia by altering normal sleep patterns and reducing REM and deeper stages of sleep. A phenomenon called *rebound insomnia* often occurs when hypnotics are withdrawn, subjecting the insomniac to very unpleasant nights of nervousness, increased difficulty falling asleep, increased intensity of dreaming, and nightmares. At this point the insomnia sufferer may assume that the pills are essential because of what happens when he or she stops taking them. The pill taking resumes and the cycle begins again.

Many poor sleepers use alcohol as a soporific. Although a small amount of alcohol may relax a physically tense person and thus help him or her to fall asleep, any amount of this particular drug will *disrupt* sleep. Sleep will tend to be nonrestorative with frequent awakenings and anxious and disturbing dreams (Hauri, 1982).

Most insomniacs who take hypnotics do so because they want to alleviate the consequences that a sleepless night has on their daytime performance. Ironically, the next morning aftereffects of hypnotics usually include drowsiness, nausea, and headache that can impair daytime functioning, mood, and performance. One newer benzodiazepine (Halcion) has a much shorter half-life than others; however, there is some indication that it may interfere with recent memory. Because the elderly often consume a variety of drugs, there are problems with toxic interaction. Changes take place in the older adult's ability to absorb, metabolize, and excrete drugs. Consequently, the toxicity profile of a particular hypnotic may be very different for the elderly than for younger adults (Scharf & Brown, 1986). Daytime complaints and health problems that occur in old age may be related to the use of sedative medications and to disorders of sleep or of the sleep-wake cycle. Chronic use of sedatives by older adults can impair their already-diminished cortical functioning. Sleep medications have been found to accumulate in the liver and kidneys and are known to depress respiratory centers, thereby raising additional questions about the safety of these drugs for elderly people, who are more likely to have impaired respiratory, hepatic, or renal functioning. Sleeping pills can also increase muscle weakness and thus increase the likelihood of falling (A. Kales & J. D. Kales, 1974; Miles & Dement, 1980).

In a prospective study of over 1 million people (Kripke, 1983), those who reported that they took sleeping medications "often" had a 50% higher mortality than those who "never" took them. These results held true even when the data were controlled for age, sex, and a history of heart disease. Those who reported "seldom" using these medications had about a 10% increased mortality. Because the elderly take far more sleeping pills than younger adults, and because the former are also more at risk for depressed breathing disorders (e.g., sleep apnea), the taking of hypnotics in old age may be fraught with greatly increased health risks (B. R. Williams, 1986).

This brief review shows that there are a number of problems with drug therapy for insomnia; the consequences of hypnotics are often more detrimental than the sleep difficulty itself. Most of the nationally known sleep researchers feel that a scientific comparison of the known risks and benefits of these compounds argues against their use except for very brief trials for acute problems (Hauri, 1982). Current medical wisdom would recommend that hypnotics be used cautiously for only short-term treatment of acute sleep problems, such as in a personal crisis, and that dosages should never be increased. It is probably also safe to use them occasionally with insomniacs to give them a night's sleep if they are having a particularly bad episode of sleeplessness or to prevent exacerbation cycles. Walsh, Sugerman, & Chambers (1986) suggest that the best use of hypnotics may be with healthy individuals who are experiencing transient or short-term sleep problems. A short course of hypnotics for this group may prevent the development of persistent insomnia that can arise out of sleep-related anxiety and/or conditioning. They think that hypnotic medication may be underused in this group and overused in persons with chronic insomnia. Another possible use would be in the prevention of jet lag in the person who expects to travel across several time zones. Sleeping medications should not be used for prolonged nightly help, for the elderly, for pregnant or nursing women, or for those with suspected sleep apnea (e.g., heavy snoring), liver and kidney disease, or alcohol abuse. The combination of alcohol and hypnotics is potentially lethal. If hypnotics are prescribed, short-acting benzodiazepines are the drug of choice, because they appear to develop tolerance more slowly and to be the safest (American Medical Association, 1984; Hauri, 1982). The recipient should be informed that the prescription is to be used only for a brief time with no increase in dosage. Sleep medication users should also be warned that they may experience some increase in sleeplessness when the pills are discontinued.

Probably the most important disadvantage of the use of hypnotics to assuage sleep disturbance is that this intervention mode prevents insomnia sufferers from developing their own personal competence in managing sleep. Attribution theorists believe that self-attributed behavior change will be maintained longer than change that is thought to be the result of an external factor such as drugs (Bootzin & Nicassio, 1978). For example, Davison, Tsujimoto, and Glaros (1973) treated college student insomniacs with a combination package of sleep medication, relaxation, and sleep scheduling. Half of those who improved were told that they had received a therapeutic dose of the drug; the other half were told that they had received an ineffective amount. Those who thought they had received the subtherapeutic pill dosage were then free to attribute their improvement to their own efforts. This group maintained their level of improvement after the drug was withdrawn. Those who thought they had received the optimum drug dosage returned to baseline levels of sleep disturbance when medication was discontinued. Unfortunately, those insomniacs who take sleep medications are likely to attribute any alleviation of their sleep problems to the drugs and therefore be unwilling to give them up.

A NONDRUG ALTERNATIVE

Because of the long-term ineffectiveness and the serious negative side effects of sleep medication, scientists have sought nondrug alternatives for the treatment of persistent insomnia. Behavioral techniques have received the most attention as a different method for the alleviation of this serious disorder. Inherent in this approach are a number of assumptions: (a) insomnia is a behavioral disorder and as such is governed by the principles of learning and conditioning; (b) insomnia is not only a symptom but is also a serious disorder in its own right that merits therapeutic intervention; and (c) clients are able to learn to cope with or to control their insomnia through the systematic application of behavioral principles (Nicassio & Buchanan, 1981). There is now about a 20-year history of research on the applications of various behavioral approaches to insomnia. Although a great deal is now known, much more knowledge needs to be developed. In chapter 4, the primary competing theories and the treatments that have evolved from them will be described and evaluated. Later chapters will present the therapeutic approach we have developed in our research program. But first the reader will need to learn the basic facts about sleep and sleep disorders, information presented in the next 2 chapters.

Chapter 2
Basic Facts About Sleep

Before a behavior therapist can offer competent help to the individual who has sleep disturbance, the therapist will have to know the basic facts about the process of sleep. Some of the information that is available and will be of high interest to the sleep-disturbed person concerns sleep stages, sleep cycles, and circadian rhythm. Clients will also want to know what amount of sleep is necessary or desirable for them. It will be important for the therapist to know how sleep requirements and patterns change with increasing age. Finally, the competent therapist should know what everyday practices and substances can disrupt sleep. Discussion of all these topics will figure prominently in the treatment for insomnia.

Our long fascination with the process of sleep is not surprising because most of us will spend approximately one third of our lives asleep. Nevertheless, a science of sleep was not possible until 50 years ago because there was no technology with which to discern and evaluate its characteristics. Beginning in 1935, scientists were able to study the electrical patterns of the brain during sleep. The 1953 discovery (Aserinksy & Kleitman) that bursts of rapid eye movement appear during periods of the night stimulated a tremendous growth in the study of sleep processes. Today, sleep researchers use a complex technology called *polysomnography*, a term that refers to the recording of sleep-related information on a polygraph. This set of diagnostic procedures is widely regarded as the most reliable and valid measure of sleep.

The use of polysomnography allows sleep researchers to monitor continuously during sleep a minimum of three different types of electrophysiologic activity: the electroencephalogram (EEG), or electrical patterns of the brain; the electro-oculogram (EOG), or eye movements; and the electromyogram (EMG), or muscle tension. For clinical assessment of sleep disorders, polysomnography generally also includes an electrocardiogram (ECG), additional EMG measures, and recordings of airflow, respiratory effort, and blood oxygen saturation. Individuals scheduled for polysomnography usually arrive at the sleep laboratory an hour before their standard bedtime. At this time, the multiple electrodes and sensors are attached by a sleep laboratory technician who will also observe the all-night recording.

A typical night of monitoring will yield up to 1500 feet of paper with multiple tracings. These tracings will be scored by a trained technician using standard criteria that were developed by Rechtschaffen and A. Kales in 1968. The scored records will then be interpreted by a clinical polysomnographer, usually a specially certified psychologist or physician. Most often this kind of complicated assessment of sleep is carried out in the setting of a sleep laboratory that has been established and certified by the Association of Sleep Disorders Centers (ASDC). Polysomnography is a very expensive diagnostic process with the average nightly cost in 1986 estimated to be $650 (a cost largely reimbursed by insurance for clinical, though not research, evaluations). Typically, a thorough evaluation of sleep disturbance can be accomplished in one night of sleep laboratory observation. In an attempt to reduce costs and to examine sleep data obtained in the natural environment, scientists have recently developed portable polysomnography equipment that provides all-night sleep recording from the home. Data are transmitted through the telephone to a computer located at the sleep laboratory while the client sleeps in his or her own bed. Not enough is known currently about home polysomnography to compare its accuracy with observations collected in the sleep laboratory.

SLEEP STAGES

Human sleep is not just the absence of wakefulness. It is not static and constant but is an active and complex state. Falling asleep and awakening is not like turning a light bulb off and then on again. Instead, normal adults gradually move through a sequence of regularly alternating stages of sleep. The term *sleep architecture* is used to describe these various patterns or *stages* that characterize sleep. Different stages of sleep are defined by distinct patterns of electrical activity and by varying behavioral and physiological states.

Sleep is first of all divided into two broad categories: non-rapid-eye-movement (non-REM or NREM) sleep and rapid-eye-movement (REM) sleep. Sleep specialists typically divide NREM sleep into four stages: stages 1, 2, 3, and 4; stages 3 and 4 are often discussed together as *delta sleep*. These stages range from very light to very deep sleep. As a person descends more deeply into sleep, the EEG goes from a fast but weak pattern to slower but stronger waves.

Stage 1 represents the lightest level of sleep and it marks the transition from wakefulness to sleep. In normal sleepers, this stage can range from 30 seconds to about 7 minutes. Reaction to outside stimuli diminishes, thoughts start to drift, and short dreamlike experiences may occur. If asked at the time, many people, especially poor sleepers, will report that they were awake during stage 1. Stage 2 sleep is the first level that sleep researchers generally agree represents true sleep. The EEG is characterized by the appearance of *sleep spindles*, or bursts of 12 to 14 distinct and highly rhythmic EEG peaks and valleys per second, and by *K-complexes*, or sudden, high-amplitude bipolar spikes. Some researchers believe that K-complexes are sleep-preserving responses to sounds in the environment. Traditionally, sleep researchers have used the first sleep spindle or K-complex as the objective marker for the onset of sleep. If awakened at this point, most people will report having been asleep. They usually do not recall any dreams though they may remember some fragments of thoughts.

Hauri and Olmstead (1983) reported that when researchers use the traditional criterion of the first sleep spindle or K-complex of stage 2, good sleepers are fairly accurate in subjectively estimating their sleep onset. For 10 good sleepers, these researchers found that the subjective estimate and the EEG-defined measure of sleep onset differed by less than 2 minutes across 3 nights of measurement. However, using this same EEG criterion, a group of 38 insomniacs subjectively overestimated the time it took them to fall asleep by 10 to 20 minutes across 3 nights. Hauri and Olmstead speculated that for poor sleepers the experience of sleep onset actually occurs at a later time during the EEG-assessed transition from sleeping to waking. They noted that insomniacs often show frequent alternations between stage 2 and wakefulness around the time of sleep onset.

Hauri and Olmstead then used a more conservative EEG criterion of sleep onset: elapsed time from lights out to the beginning of the first 15 minutes of *solid* sleep. That is, these 15 minutes are not interrupted by any awakenings or by reversals to stage 1. Using this marker, they found that the poor sleepers were able to estimate sleep onset about as accurately as the good sleepers could using the more traditional criterion. Hauri and Olmstead suggest that because of poor sleepers' frequent stage reversals during the early part of sleep, the traditional EEG markers of sleep onset are not appropriate for them. Coates et al. (1982) also found significant differences between insomniacs' subjective estimates of sleep onset latency and EEG stage 1 sleep but not between self-report and NREM stage 2 sleep. During sleep onset, the insomniac appears to experience frequent alternations between stage 2 and wakefulness. A number of studies lend corroboration by finding that insomniacs usually report mental activity or being awake when aroused during stage 1, and about half the time during the early part of stage 2.

The main characteristic of REM sleep is the rapid eye movements that give it its name. Even though closed, the eyes periodically dart vertically and horizontally. In this stage, a person is clearly asleep but the EEG looks like that of someone who is awake, as though the sleeper were actively thinking. On the EEG, REM sleep is seen as a low-voltage, mixed-frequency pattern. The EEG resembles that of stage 1 but with more of a sawtooth appearance. If awakened during REM sleep, 80% of people will report full-fledged, vivid dreams. Only about 5% will report dreams in NREM awakenings (Dement & Kleitman, 1957). REM sleep has some of the characteristics of lighter sleep and some of deeper sleep; as such, it cannot be easily classified on this dimension.

The body appears to require REM sleep, and if prevented from getting it on one night, the body will recapture it another night. People who are deprived of REM sleep on one night will experience *REM rebound* the next night. The rebound effect means that much more time will be spent in REM sleep on the subsequent night, resulting in frequent dreams. When the REM deprivation is long term, the dreams often take on a nightmarish quality. The most frequent cause of REM deprivation is the use of hypnotic sleep medication (see chapter 1). During a REM period, there is near paralysis of many large muscles, although the smaller muscles may twitch from time to time. This pattern may be designed to protect sleep by preventing the acting out of movements from dreams.

Some theorists posit a sleep system that regulates the different states of wakefulness and sleep. The reticular activating system (RAS) may be primarily responsible for the regulation of the condition of wakefulness, whereas the serotonergic sleep system may control the condition of sleep. Quiet wakefulness and perhaps even stage 1 transition sleep may be produced by low RAS activity. However, the sleep system may have to be activated in order to induce stage 2 and delta sleep. The process of sleep probably requires the harmonious integration of these two systems (Hauri, 1982).

SLEEP CYCLES

During normal sleep, individuals move back and forth among the four stages of sleep, interspersed with brief awakenings. Although this process is actually distributed on a continuum, sleep researchers have agreed upon criteria that mark the beginnings and ends of the various stages. This sequence of moving through the sleep stages is referred to as a sleep *cycle*. Figure 2.1 taken from Hauri (1982), illustrates a typical pattern of sleep cycles for a young, adult good sleeper. The process starts with a brief period, perhaps 5 minutes, of relaxed but drowsy wakefulness in which the EEG shows alpha waves when the eyes are closed. The next 1 to 5 minutes are spent passing through stage 1, becoming more and more relaxed, with thoughts beginning to drift off. During about the next 20 minutes, the good sleeper descends deeper into sleep within stage 2. The sleeper is definitely asleep and any thinking that occurs is fragmented. By about 15 to 30 minutes into the sleep process, our subject enters delta sleep or deep sleep, typically lasting 30 to 60 minutes. At this point the good sleeper ascends back to stage 2, during which time a first, brief (about 5 minutes) REM period will occur. This short REM experience yields back to stage 2, an event that marks the beginning of the second sleep cycle. The first cycle lasted about 90 minutes. The typical sleeper will go through 4 to 6 of these cycles per night.

Examination of Figure 2.1 reveals that each sleep cycle is not an exact repetition of the sequence of the first cycle but has its own distinct combination of the various sleep stages. For example, after the first sleep cycle, delta sleep is confined to 2 or 3 additional brief (5 to 10 minutes) periods during the first half of the night and is rarely seen during the second half of the night. REM and stage 2 sleep alternate in cycles of about 90 minutes in adults. However, most of REM sleep occurs in the second half of the night. REM periods lengthen to an average of about 20 to 30 minutes and become much more intense.

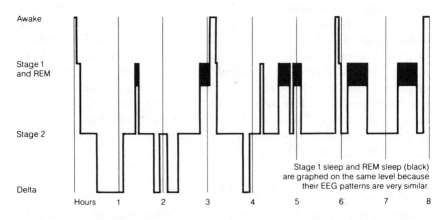

FIGURE 2.1. Typical Sleep Pattern of a Young Human Adult

Note: From Hauri, P. (1982). *The sleep disorders* (p. 8) by P. Hauri, 1982, Kalamazoo, MI: Scope Publications, the Upjohn Company. Copyright 1982 by Peter Hauri and the Upjohn Company. Reprinted with permission.

Several times during the night a person will surface to full wakefulness for several minutes, even though he or she may not remember such events the next morning.

On a typical night, a young, adult good sleeper will spend about 5% of the time in stage 1, about 50% in stage 2, and 20% in delta or deep sleep. REM sleep will comprise about 25% of the night (Youkilis & Bootzin, 1981). Under normal circumstances the body will get the amount of sleep it needs and will on the average distribute it in these amounts across the various stages. However, there is no fixed amount of sleep that meets the needs of each person. Individuals have to find out what amount is appropriate for them by the way they feel and perform the next day. With increasing age there is a widespread tendency to sleep less deeply and for shorter periods. Many older adults who complain of not getting 8 hours of sleep do not realize that sleeping needs and patterns often change with advancing age. At this time, it is unclear if older people need less sleep or are simply unable to obtain as much sleep as before (Miles & Dement, 1980).

The entire physiology of a person alters during movement back and forth through the sleep states. Cardiac rate, respiration, cerebral blood flow, acid secretion, blood pressure, and muscle tone are just a few of the functions that are affected by the waking, NREM, and REM cycling. In general NREM sleep is consistently quiet from a physiological standpoint. Cardiac, respiration, temperature, and blood pressure rates are all very regular and reach their lowest levels for the day. In REM sleep, however, physiology fluctuates considerably and has some unique aspects as well. In some individuals, these systems may work normally when they are awake, but malfunction during sleep. For example, a person may have normal respiration while awake but demonstrate dangerous and potentially lethal breathing lapses while asleep.

CIRCADIAN RHYTHM

For most people the cycle of sleep-wake alternation takes about 24 hours to complete and is linked to the presence or absence of sunlight. Sleep is best during dark hours and peak alertness occurs when the sun is up. Other bodily functions also follow this diurnal rhythm. For example, body temperature is lowest during nighttime sleep, rises as morning approaches, and is highest during the day. However, there is a good deal of individual variation in the point at which optimum efficiency is reached. The terms "early bird" or "lark" and "night owl" describe those who reach their peaks at different points in the day (Hauri, 1982).

When humans are deprived of such cues as clocks and a view of the outdoors, they may eventually drift to a somewhat longer circadian cycle, perhaps as long as 28 hours. A few may even develop much longer cycles. Some individuals, even when the usual cues are present, demonstrate circadian rhythm difficulties with their sleep. It is not unusual for insomniacs who struggle to get 8 hours of sleep to alter their circadian rhythm by sleeping late in the morning and taking naps. In this case, sleep experts believe that the best way to resynchronize circadian rhythm is to have a regular wake-up time each day. This tactic is best because individuals are usually able to bring waking-up time under voluntary control through practices like using an alarm clock and taking a morning shower. It would be much harder to put falling asleep time under voluntary control because individuals usually cannot force themselves to fall asleep on demand (Hauri, 1982).

SLEEP REQUIREMENTS

How much sleep does a person need to be alert and energetic throughout the day? The consensus in our society is that the optimum amount of sleep is 8 hours. There is some truth to this belief. Numerous surveys have shown that the average amount of sleep obtained by adults in the United States is between 7 and 8 hours. About 50% of a sample of 4000 college freshmen in Florida averaged 7.5 to 8.5 hours of sleep per night. This average amount of sleep has been found in a wide variety of settings, such as in northern latitudes where the ratio of light to darkness shifts radically during different times of the year, and in experimental settings where access to clocks and sunlight is removed (Webb & Agnew, 1975).

However, these figures are *average* amounts of sleep and they are not optimum for everyone, as is widely believed. Many people require shorter or longer amounts of sleep but worry needlessly because their sleep pattern does not match the magical 8-hour standard. In fact, insomnia can develop from performance anxiety over not getting the "correct" amount of sleep. Sometimes, naturally long sleepers have pressure put on them to sleep less because sleeping more than 8 hours connotes laziness. Normal sleep across individuals may be in the range of 3 to 10 hours per night. Each man and woman, adult and child has a personal ideal amount of sleep. Even within an individual, however, this optimal amount may be compromised with age, physical and emotional health, lifestyle, and societal demands. For example, women who work full-time get less sleep than those who have part-time jobs; rotating-shift workers get less sleep than day-shift workers (American Medical Association, 1984). As a society, we are probably somewhat sleep-deprived. School children in 1900 got about an hour more sleep per night than children of the same age in the 1960s. College students now sleep about 1.5 hours less per night than they did in 1910 but many wish to sleep longer (Webb & Agnew, 1975). Many people complain that they do not have enough hours in the day to do all the things they need to or want to accomplish and so they stay up longer than they might otherwise. Webb and Agnew suggest that in a modern society there are many contributors to chronic sleep deprivation: rigid work schedules, increased opportunities for nighttime social activities, television, and the invention of electric lights that allow people to read at night.

SLEEP AND THE OLDER ADULT

The sleep of the older adult is different in many ways from that of younger individuals. In fact, the physiology of sleep changes gradually across the entire developmental span. Total sleep time decreases as a person grows older. A newborn sleeps about 18 hours out of every 24 and this amount drops to 10 to 12 hours by age 4 and to around 9 or 10 hours at age 10. Experts think that the optimum sleep pattern is achieved at about the age of 10. Most children of this age fall asleep easily and rapidly at about the same time each day, sleep soundly, and are completely alert for the rest of the day. By adolescence, the average amount of time spent in sleep drops steeply to about 7.5 to 8 hours (although this figure may represent less sleep time than is optimal for individuals). From that age there is a very gradual decline in amount of sleep to 6.5 hours for older adults (Hauri, 1982). Although time asleep decreases over the years, time spent in bed *increases* after about age 40, resulting in a decrease of sleep efficiency. Sleep efficiency is the ratio of amount of sleep obtained divided by amount of time in bed. Older people spend more time in bed but get less sleep. Some older adults maintain the amount of sleep they have been accustomed to in earlier years by regular napping.

The sleep architecture of the older person is also unlike that of those who are younger. Characteristically the elderly will experience decreases in the periods of deeper sleep, or delta stage sleep, and will experience increases in light sleep, or stages 1 and 2. At age 70, the delta stage makes up less than 10% of the night's sleep, compared with 15% to 25% during adolescence and younger adulthood (Walsh, 1983). As a result of this greater percentage of light sleep, older adults also find themselves awakening many more times during the night.

With age there is not only a decrease in amount of sleep and a change in kind of sleep but also an increase in sleep disturbances. Among children, sleep disturbances tend to be concentrated among night terrors, enuresis, and bedtime fears. Adolescents typically are sleep deprived and have difficulty getting up in the mornings. For the elderly, there is a steep increase in the incidence of sleep apnea, nocturnal myoclonus, and insomnia. Regarding insomnia, older adults suffer more from frequent and longer nighttime awakenings or too early awakenings, whereas the younger person with insomnia will typically complain of trouble getting to sleep. All of these changes appear to occur earlier in females than in males (Dement, 1983).

These changes in sleep for the older adult are well documented both in sleep laboratories and by self-report. However, there is less agreement as to the cause of these changes. Are these alterations in sleep a part of the normal developmental or aging process or is there an increase in sleep pathology that is age related? Is there a decrease in the need for sleep or are older adults less able to get the sleep that they need? Do the increases in health problems found in older adults contribute to their sleep problems? Or can these changes be explained fully by the altered lifestyle of the elderly?

Most sleep experts would probably feel that a combination of all these factors contributes to the changes in older sleep. Regestein (1980) presents one of the fullest discussions of this issue. First, he feels that sleep laboratory research shows a definite decrease in the soundness of the sleep of older adults due to degenerative nervous system changes. Less sound sleep renders the older person more vulnerable to disruption of sleep from other sources such as noise, caffeine intake, or worry about lack of sleep. However, not all older adults demonstrate this degeneration, just as not all of this age group show sleep disturbance.

Second, older adults do have more physical illness than those who are younger. For example, many of them suffer from arthritis that can produce sufficient nighttime pain to disrupt sleep. Other diseases or disorders are treated with prescription medications that can interfere with sleep. A common drug for the treatment of asthma contains adrenaline; diuretics are often prescribed for hypertension and if taken at night may lead to frequent arousals to urinate (Bootzin, Engle-Friedman, & Hazelwood, 1983).

Third, older adults have more of a tendency to alter their circadian rhythm. They may be isolated from steady contact with other people. If they no longer work, there is less reason for them to get up at the same time every morning or to keep some kind of regular schedule. Regular napping can steadily push bedtime to a later and later hour. All of these practices can result eventually in a reversal of days and nights or to no correlation between the older adult's sleep time and that engaged in by most of the rest of the population. The resulting fragmented and off-schedule sleep may very well be labeled as insomnia by themselves and others.

Furthermore, the elderly frequently reduce their level of physical activity and lead relatively sedentary lives. New stresses present themselves in the form of financial worries, the illness or death of a spouse or of close friends, loneliness, loss of self-esteem, reduction in physical and intellectual abilities, and curtailment of usual interests and activities. These lifestyle changes may also influence the quality of sleep (Miles & Dement, 1980).

Finally, Lichstein and Fischer (1985) point to the general lack of public knowledge about the relationship between sleep and age as another possible culprit in the development of insomnia. Changes in sleep patterns occurring with advancing age may be an inevitable part of the aging process. If older adults are not expecting these changes and do not recognize them as part of the developmental process, then they may interpret these changes as pathological. As amount and quality of sleep decrease with advancing age, the frustrated older adult may engage in many kinds of activities designed to reestablish the previous habitual level of sleep. Unfortunately, many of these activities, such as taking sleep medications, have the paradoxical effect of further eroding the quality and quantity of sleep.

SLEEP HYGIENE

Some people sleep well under virtually all circumstances, especially those who are younger. Others may sleep well unless certain circumstances or ingested substances intervene. As people grow older, they are more likely to be vulnerable to sleep disruption from such influences. A smaller number of individuals will not sleep well even under the most ideal conditions. If a client complains of long-standing, severe insomnia, most likely that client belongs in the third category; this category includes people who have trouble sleeping regardless of the situational influences. When someone complains of mild or moderate insomnia, it is difficult to know to what extent the poor sleep is related to these outside factors. The natural changes that take place as one enters middle age may render a person especially vulnerable to sleep-disrupting effects of internal and external environmental events.

Providing oneself with an ideal set of sleep circumstances is what sleep researchers call practicing good sleep hygiene. Many attempts have been made to isolate factors that may cause or contribute to sleeping disorders. Among these factors are the sleep environment, ingested substances, sleep scheduling, presleep activities, daytime behaviors, and attitudes toward sleep. A brief background of the research basis for sleep hygiene is provided in the following pages. Specific information for the application of sleep hygiene rules to the treatment of insomnia is provided in chapter 7.

Sleep Environment

There are many factors in each person's sleep environment that may or may not be conducive to rapid onset and good quality of sleep. Examples of such factors include the level of noise and light, the firmness of the bed, the room temperature, and the presence of a bedpartner. Unfortunately, there are few set rules for prescribing a certain sleep environment for every poor sleeper. Individuals vary widely in their reactions to and their preferences for these various factors.

As an example, let us consider the noise level in the bedroom. Generally, more noise leads to delayed sleep onset, decreased depth of sleep, and poorer sleep maintenance. However, many people find that certain kinds of *white noise* (masking sounds) such as from an air conditioner or humidifier, are soothing and sleep inducing. Hauri (1982) has reviewed the literature on the effects of noise on sleep. In one study, the awakening threshold among seven college students varied from the level of a whisper to a level equivalent to that found in a disco. The more deeply asleep the person is, the more noise that is required to rouse the sleeper. Sporadic loud noises are more disruptive than constant ones. In a study of Los Angeles residents, those who lived close to the airport got an average of 45 minutes less sleep per night and less deep sleep than those who lived farther away in quieter areas. Sensitivity to noise does increase with age, and women seem more sensitive to it than do men. Because older adults have more difficulty returning to sleep once awakened, a noisy sleep environment may pose even more problems for this group.

Another example for consideration is the presence or absence of a bedpartner. Having a restless sleeping partner is likely to lower the quality of sleep. Monroe (1969) found that couples who share a bed had less deep sleep than when they slept in separate beds. A partner who snores presents a significant challenge to the poor sleeper. Yet some people may feel lonely or insecure when they are alone in bed and therefore may then sleep less well. Again we can see the importance of individual preferences in the matter of sleep environments. Another factor that has been shown to have some disruptive effect on sleep is room temperature. When the temperature goes above 75°F, humans awaken more often, move about more in their sleep, sleep less deeply, and experience less dreaming sleep (Hauri, 1982). When temperatures are too low, individuals may feel too cold to fall asleep. For most people, temperatures between 65°F and 70°F are the most comfortable for sleeping.

Sleep-Interfering Substances

The best-known facts about sleep-interfering substances concern the effects of central nervous system stimulants. Of special concern are the nighttime ingestion of caffeine in beverages, food, or medications for pain or to control weight or allergy symptoms. Caffeine is a very potent arousal drug, much more so than most people realize. It is well established as a powerful sleep disruptor even in those people who would argue that caffeine has no impact on their sleep. For example, one study showed that 2 cups of a beverage containing caffeine prior to bedtime produced changes in most standard EEG sleep parameters; 4 cups heightened these effects (Karacan et al., 1976a). In terms of laboratory-verified sleep onset latency, mean values for 18 volunteers were 11 minutes at baseline, 21 minutes after 2 cups of coffee, and 32 minutes after 4 cups. Those who received a 4-cup equivalent dose of caffeine took 28 minutes to fall asleep. Eliminating caffeine in 10 psychiatric inpatients reduced the number of awakenings and also reduced the requests for sleep medication (Edelstein, Keaton-Brasted, & Burg, 1984). The maximal blood concentrations for caffeine are reached within one hour, and its half-life is at least 3.5 hours. Therefore, caffeine ingested an hour before bedtime is likely to cause problems getting to sleep, whereas caffeine taken at bedtime may result in unwelcome middle-of-the-night awakenings (Karacan et al., 1976a). It is true that some individuals are more sensitive to the effects of stimulants than are others.

Most of our clients know about the arousal properties of caffeine. However, many of them only give lip service to the need to curtail their use of this drug. In our work we have also found inconsistent knowledge among insomniacs about what substances do or do not contain caffeine. Those beverages that contain caffeine include regular coffee, regular tea and some herb teas, hot chocolate, regular cola soft drinks, and the specific soft drinks Dr. Pepper, Mountain Dew, Mr. Pibb, and Mellow Yellow. The chief foods that have caffeine are anything containing chocolate. Over-the-counter medications with caffeine or another stimulant include Excedrin, Midol, Dristan cold remedy, Sudafed decongestant, Dexatrim diet pills, Aqua-Ban diuretic, No-Doz — and many more. Also, many prescription drugs have stimulant properties, such as drugs that are used to treat asthma and migraine headaches. Other potential sources of stimulants are amphetamines, steroids, adrenergic blockers, and bronchodilators. Substances that do not ordinarily have caffeine are decaffeinated coffee or tea, many but not all herb teas, 7-Up and Sprite soft drinks, root beer, ginger ale, decaffeinated colas, and plain aspirin or Tylenol.

Nicotine is another central nervous system stimulant that is related to difficulty falling asleep (J. D. Kales et al., 1984). In a study of chronic smokers, Soldatos, J. D. Kales, Scharf, Bixler, & A. Kales (1980) found that the latency to fall asleep in the sleep laboratory was 44 minutes for a group of smokers (average of 1.25 packs per day) and 30 minutes for 50 matched nonsmokers. Sleep also showed significant improvement when nicotine use was eliminated. When a smaller sample of 8 smokers (average of 2 packs per day) were asked to give up smoking, their average sleep onset latency decreased from 52 minutes per night to 34 minutes after only 4 days of abstinence from nicotine. Four subjects who continued to abstain from smoking showed additional improved sleep onset. Little change was noted on other sleep parameters between smokers and nonsmokers.

It is paradoxical that sleep medications and alcohol, two categories of substances that are often taken to benefit sleep, actually interfere with good sleep. The sleep-interfering properties of hypnotics were detailed in chapter 1. After a brief period of efficacy, hypnotics can begin to *cause* sleep disturbance by altering normal sleep patterns and by reducing dreaming and deep sleep periods. When taken in moderate amounts, alcohol does relax a person and may facilitate falling asleep in an overly tense person. However, alcohol, a central nervous system depressant, leads later in the night to decreased dreaming and deep sleep, to more fitful sleep, and to frequent awakenings so that the person does not feel refreshed the next morning (Hauri, 1982; Maxmen, 1981).

Sleep Scheduling

Many normally good sleepers have found themselves unaccountably unable to fall asleep at their usual time on Sunday night. It is likely that the majority of these "Sunday-night insomniacs" went to sleep much later than usual on Saturday night and then slept late on Sunday and/or took a Sunday afternoon nap. Consequently, their bodies are not ready for sleep at the regular time on Sunday night. Most of these individuals will arise at their typical time on Monday morning and go to work feeling a little draggy. By Monday night they are tired, fall asleep easily, and get right back into their usual pattern of good sleeping.

The insomnia sufferer, however, in response to poor sleep, may develop an irregular pattern of sleeping across the entire week. The poor sleeper often sleeps in after an unsatisfactory night and takes one or more naps each day, all in an attempt to get a total of 8 hours of rest. On the evening following a poor night's sleep he or she may go to bed early, feeling tired though not really sleepy. Unfortunately, these attempts to get sleep usually cause disruptions in the sleep-wake rhythm that have the opposite effect of leading to more problems with sleep. For example, going to sleep early because it takes so long to get to sleep will probably result in a longer period to fall asleep because the person was not drowsy to begin with. Also, there can develop an unusual pattern of sleeping times that interfere with work, family activities, and social life. The combination of reduced need for sleep and increased difficulty with sleep often leads the elderly to go to bed very early and then be awake from 3 a.m. on, so that their awake schedule does not match that of the rest of the world.

Our bodies respond best to a relatively consistent timetable. Going to sleep and getting up at around the same time each day and not taking naps will result in sounder sleep. The time when this sleep period takes place and the amount of sleep are not so important and are individual matters; what matters most is its consistency from day to day. Regularity of sleep scheduling is even more crucial for someone who suffers from insomnia.

Presleep Activities

In general, the hour before bedtime should be one in which the potential sleeper prepares for sleep. Most of us think of this period as a time to wind down in anticipation of getting into bed and falling asleep rapidly. This hour serves as a transition period between the waking of the day and the sleep of the night. Those of us who are parents usually recognize this need for a transition period for our young children and provide them with a regular nighttime routine of bath, story, favorite stuffed animal, and lullaby. Adults have the same need for a transition period. Most of us cannot go abruptly from waking to sleeping. Presleep activities often involve some kind of relaxation, a putting aside of the troubles of the day just past and of the day to come, and a set of presleep routines. Very busy, somewhat obsessive poor sleepers report that the only time they have to worry about their day is at bedtime. We encourage them to schedule a definite time each day, preferably not even near bedtime, to do this kind of worrying. Another common and disruptive kind of worry is that of not being able to fall asleep. A large majority of insomniacs engage in this kind of presleep activity almost every night. Discussion of sleep hygiene should always include this topic and help in eliminating it. For a more detailed discussion see the section in chapter 4 on performance anxiety.

One of my psychotherapy clients began to experience difficulty falling asleep near the end of her treatment for nonsleep problems. A brief discussion of her presleep activities revealed that she had been engaging very successfully in a set of winding-down practices from 8 to 9 p.m. each evening and became very drowsy and ready for sleep. Recently, however, she had begun to use the subsequent hour to set out her clothes and work papers for the next day and to plan what she had to do at her office. This set of practices aroused her, she became very alert, and when she got into bed at 10 o'clock, she was no longer drowsy and could not fall asleep. Fortunately, she told me of the problem before it had existed for very long. I was able to recommend that she reverse the way she was spending these two prebedtime hours, and her problem disappeared within a matter of days. If she had not received this simple advice and had continued to experience trouble falling asleep, she would have been a prime candidate to develop performance anxiety and perhaps to promote a temporary sleep problem into chronic insomnia.

Another helpful presleep activity is the development of a set of prebedtime routines that are engaged in every night in as close to the same order as possible. This routine usually involves such behaviors as walking the dog, turning out the lights, locking the door, checking on the children, brushing teeth, setting the alarm, arranging favorite pillows in the preferred positions, and others. Some sleep researchers include these routines under the category of sleep hygiene, whereas others include them as part of the stimulus control treatment. Because presleep routines help to signal that bedtime has arrived, I have also discussed them in more detail as part of stimulus control techniques later.

Daytime Behaviors

Many of the behaviors that we engage in during the day can influence the quality and quantity of our sleep at night. Probably the most important daytime behavior that affects sleep is regular exercise. Research on chronic insomniacs indicates that they may lead more sedentary daytime lives and be less fit than good sleepers (de la Peña, 1978; Marchini, Coates, Magistad, & Waldum, 1983). Other studies have shown that a steady habit of physical exercise is conducive to greater amounts of the night spent in deep sleep which is more restorative sleep (Baekeland & Lasky, 1966). Better muscle tone evidently promotes muscular relaxation when the body is at rest. Occasional exercise, however, does not have this beneficial effect. Morning exercise aids sleep less than activity in the late afternoon or early evening (Horne & Porter, 1976). Exercise at night is likely to stimulate the person and delay sleep onset.

Another daytime behavior that can have adverse effects on sleep is weight loss. Higher caloric intake is associated with long and uninterrupted sleep while lower caloric levels are associated with short and fragmented sleep especially in the second half of the night. Some researchers have explained this phenomenon as related to survival — a hungry animal needs to be awake and foraging, but those that are not hungry are safest if they hide and sleep. Others attribute the fragmented sleep more simply to awakening from the signals of pangs of hunger. Insomniacs who suffer only from delayed sleep onset and do not report being hungry at bedtime need not worry about the issue of amount and timing of caloric intake. However, those poor sleepers who awake in the middle of the night or too early in the morning and who are on restricted caloric intake can try a prebedtime snack with calories saved from earlier in the day. Some researchers recommend a combination of carbohydrates and protein, such as cheese and crackers or milk and a graham cracker (Hauri, 1982). It is also important to note that a full meal stimulates digestive activity that can interfere with sleep. It is best to eat dinner several hours before bedtime.

Knowledge and Practice of Sleep Hygiene

Although most sleep researchers consider adherence to sleep hygiene principles to be important, little is known about the overall sleep hygiene awareness and practices of either good sleepers or insomniacs. From our experience, many insomniacs claim to have sophisticated knowledge of these factors and to be faithful practitioners of good sleep hygiene behavior. In recent years, there has been a great deal of media publicity about sleep hygiene. Insomniacs, by virtue of their special personal interest in this topic, are likely to be avid consumers of such information. Whether they put such knowledge into consistent practice, however, is open to question because they continue to have sleep difficulties.

Investigation of these issues has been hampered by the absence of a sleep hygiene scale. We undertook to develop such a scale to use in our research and treatment efforts. The Sleep Hygiene Awareness and Practice Scale (SHAPS) has three parts: (a) general knowledge of what specific activities are beneficial, disruptive, or have no effect on sleep; (b) knowledge of what substances contain caffeine; and (c) typical practice of those behaviors that benefit or disrupt sleep. This scale will be presented in chapter 5. In a study of 44 sleep onset insomniacs, 49 sleep maintenance insomniacs, and 50 good sleepers (Lacks & Rotert, 1986), poor sleepers did have more sleep hygiene knowledge than good sleepers, but practiced it less often. Sleep onset insomniacs and sleep maintenance insomniacs had equivalent hygiene awareness, but the fomer group had less healthy hygiene practices. Among insomniacs, there was almost perfect recognition of the effects of caffeine in disrupting sleep. In spite of this awareness, however, poor sleepers continued to drink caffeinated beverages 1 or 2 nights a week and to have some deficiencies in their knowledge of which substances contain this stimulant. Hygiene knowledge was most deficient on the effects of nicotine, sleep medication, alcohol, and exercise. Hygiene practice needed most attention in the areas of regular exercise, prebedtime relaxation, and managing prebedtime worry.

It is hard to know which comes first, poor sleep or poor sleep hygiene. Poor sleep may lead to an increase in undesirable habits such as heavy caffeine use, variable bedtimes, naps, and sleep medications. These practices in turn lead to worse sleep and so on. Although the results suggest that poor sleep hygiene is not a primary cause of insomnia for most poor sleepers, we recommend that behavior therapists continue to address this element in their therapy to help poor sleepers avoid exacerbation cycles. Use of the SHAPS during screening would aid the therapist by showing areas in which each individual might profit by education and/or exhortation.

Chapter 3
Sleep Disorders

Careful categorization of the client's sleep problem will be essential to the selection of the most appropriate therapy. Not all forms of sleep disturbance are amenable to behavioral treatment. In fact, some forms of insomnia are indicative of organic sleep disorders that require medical intervention and one of these diagnoses can indicate the presence of a life-threatening condition. This chapter will describe the various sleep disorders and indicate desirable treatment interventions.

As more researchers and clinicians have become interested in sleep disturbances, specialized centers for their study and treatment have proliferated, primarily in major medical centers and hospitals. To ensure high standards among these centers, the Association of Sleep Disorders Centers (ASDC) was founded in 1975. This group certifies centers and maintains professional standards for their operation. In 1986, there were 68 certified sleep disorders centers in the United States and Canada.

When the ASDC was founded, a number of diagnostic schemes were in use to categorize sleep disorders. One of the early achievements of the ASDC was to establish an official nosology of sleep and arousal disorders. Since this diagnostic system was published (Association of Sleep Disorders Centers, 1979), it has shown promise of being widely accepted as the standard nomenclature. One sign of its acceptance was its inclusion as an appendix to the third edition of the American Psychiatric Association's *Diagnostic and Statistical Manual of Mental Disorders* (*DSM III* 1980). As with other kinds of disorders, the differential diagnosis of sleep disturbances is essential for making appropriate treatment decisions.

The ASDC system is based upon the chief complaint of the client (e.g., trouble getting to sleep vs. daytime sleepiness). Sleep is a finely regulated and highly sensitive system. It depends on many environmental and psychological factors as well as on the integrity of the body's biological systems. Given such a complex process, it is not surprising

33

that there are numerous conditions that can throw off the smooth running of this system. A great deal of the information in this chapter was gleaned from the ASDC descriptions (Association of Sleep Disorders Centers, 1979). Clinicians who expect to treat insomniacs should become familiar with this diagnostic system. Chapter 5 will deal with the process of making the differential diagnosis through questionnaires and interview.

ASDC nosology recognizes four major categories of sleep disturbance, each of which has a number of subtypes:

- Disorders of Initiating and Maintaining Sleep (DIMS).
- Disorders of Excessive Somnolence (DOES).
- Disorders of the Sleep-Wake Schedule.
- Disorders Associated with Sleep, Sleep Stages, or Partial Arousals (Parasomnias).

DISORDERS OF INITIATING AND MAINTAINING SLEEP (DIMS)

The clinician who works with clients who complain of insomnia will be confronted primarily with DIMS diagnoses. Therefore, I have chosen to emphasize the diagnosis of this kind of sleep disorder and have only briefly described the other 3 categories. Individuals suffering from the three other major types of sleep disorders are more likely to present themselves for help at sleep disorders centers than to seek out the services of a behavior therapist. The Disorders of Initiating and Maintaining Sleep diagnoses are made up of those disturbances that have traditionally been labeled as insomnia. It is a heterogeneous group of conditions; however, the unifying factor is that all are thought to result in disturbed sleep or in diminished sleep. Although the term insomnia describes the final common pathway of sleeplessness, there are many diverse sources, both physical and psychological, leading to this end product. These diverse sources are represented by the 9 subcategories of DIMS that are listed in Table 3.1.

Psychophysiological DIMS

The first subcategory within DIMS is psychophysiological DIMS, which can be further subdivided into either of two patterns: (a) transient and situational, or (b) persistent. It can be characterized by difficulty falling asleep or remaining asleep, premature morning awakening, or any combination of these three. The sleep disturbance must be verified objectively in the sleep laboratory. Individuals who

Table 3.1. Disorders of Initiating and Maintaining Sleep: Subtypes from the Diagnostic
Classification System of the Association of Sleep Disorders Centers

Disorders of Initiating and Maintaining Sleep (DIMS)

1. Psychophysiological DIMS
2. DIMS Associated with Psychiatric Disorders
3. DIMS Associated with the Use of Drugs and Alcohol
4. DIMS Associated with Sleep-Induced Respiratory Impairment
5. DIMS Associated with Nocturnal Myoclonus and "Restless Legs"
6. DIMS Associated with Other Medical, Toxic, and Environmental Conditions
7. Childhood-Onset DIMS
8. DIMS Associated with Other Conditions
9. No DIMS Abnormality

suffer from this type of DIMS generally will not complain of being sleepy during the day but instead will say that they are tired, irritable, and lacking in energy and motivation to perform their daytime activities. Often this type of DIMS is diagnosed by excluding other categories, such as sleep disturbance associated with serious medical or psychiatric problems.

Transient and situational psychophysiological DIMS refers to a brief period of disturbed sleep usually provoked by some acute emotional event or by a personal crisis or perceived threat. Examples of such events are a death in the family, divorce, hospitalization, and loss of a job. To earn this diagnosis, the disturbed sleep may not last longer than 3 weeks after the end of the precipitating event. Almost all people will experience transient sleep disturbance at a few points in their lives; however, the ASDC description states that those people who are insecure and who have a low threshold for emotional arousal are most vulnerable to this disruption. The key to the transient diagnosis will often be a sudden and sharp episode of sleeplessness. However, sudden onset of sleep problems may also be seen at the beginning of serious psychiatric disturbance or some medical conditions, such as metabolic disturbance.

If the poor sleep lasts longer than the 3 weeks, it is classified as persistent although sleep researchers often use a more conservative criterion, such as 6 months. Even if this type of insomnia may have started in a crisis period, it now functions autonomously. Persistent psychophysiological DIMS is viewed as the result of a chronic, somatized tension-anxiety and negative conditioning of sleep. Often these disturbed sleepers are habitually tense, rigid, obsessive, and restless individuals who have multiple somatic complaints, such as tension and headaches. Their symptoms are not serious enough, however, to warrant a psychiatric diagnosis. These people ofter refer to themselves as "light" sleepers. A typical pattern is that as sleep problems begin, apprehension about the loss of sleep leads this kind of person to strive harder to sleep and in the process to develop performance anxiety toward sleep. These individuals will often fall asleep when they are not trying to, such as when watching television or reading. Or they may paradoxically sleep well in the sleep laboratory, a somewhat opposite pattern from good sleepers, because they enter that situation not expecting to get a good night of sleep. After some time with this pattern, the poor sleeper may develop conditioned negative attitudes and behaviors associated with the bed and bedroom. The bed becomes a conditioned cue for wakefulness instead of sleepiness. These people then will sleep better away from home, for example in a hotel. More information on personality styles of insomniacs, performance anxiety, and conditioning will be found in chapter 4.

If psychophysiological DIMS is identified during the transient stage, many clinicians believe that a brief, time-limited course of hypnotic medication may be the treatment of choice. Because only a few nights of medication are given, tolerance cannot be established and normal sleep patterns will not be seriously compromised. The chief advantage of this type of intervention is that it may prevent the development of conditioning cycles that can turn situational DIMS into a lifelong problem. If this kind of DIMS becomes persistent, the optimum strategy will be behavioral techniques to combat the high tension, faulty habits, and conditioning (Hauri, 1982).

DIMS Associated with Psychiatric Disorders

The most frequent psychiatric disorders associated with DIMS are anxiety, depression, and schizophrenia. In these cases, sleep problems typically wax and wane in conjunction with the presence or absence of the psychiatric symptoms; in psychophysiological DIMS the sleeplessness persists consistently across time. The more typical pattern for the anxious client will be lengthened sleep onset. However, with primary depression, sleep onset is generally left undisturbed while sleep maintenance and early-morning-awakening problems are common. Even though depressives may sleep more than usual, they wake up complaining of feeling tired and unrefreshed. In unipolar depression, EEG patterns reveal long and intensive REM sleep earlier than usual in the night and reduced delta or deep sleep. The severity of depression and the severity of insomnia are often strongly correlated.

The schizophrenic may suffer from long sleep latency periods (due to extreme anxiety and preoccupation) but once asleep is able to stay asleep for up to 7 or 8 hours. This pattern will result in the patient's awakening later and later in the day, culminating in a partial or complete inversion of the day-night sleep cycle. Schizophrenics may also experience vivid dreaming of implausible, bizarre, hostile, or anxious content. For the subcategory of sleep disturbance associated with psychiatric disorders the best approach is to treat the underlying psychopathology. Behavioral approaches may be a useful adjunct to the primary treatment; however, the effectiveness of such a combined approach has not yet been empirically verified.

DIMS associated with the Use of Drugs and Alcohol

Many kinds of drugs can cause sleep disturbance. Certain patterns of disrupted sleep will be present during use of these drugs while other patterns appear while the drug is being withdrawn. Specific problems can include tolerance to or withdrawal from CNS depressants, sustained use of CNS stimulants, sustained use of or withdrawal from other drugs, and chronic alcoholism. Some of these sleep-disturbing drugs may have been prescribed for legitimate medical problems like asthma, cancer, seizures, and thyroid dysfunction.

One of the most frequent drug problems seen by clinicians is the prolonged use of hypnotics with the concomitant development of tolerance, dependence, disruption of natural sleep patterns, and REM suppression with rebound upon withdrawal from the drug (see chapter 1). Many users of these drugs were first introduced to their nightly use during a routine hospitalization even though they may not have demonstrated any sleep problems at that time. Others developed dependence upon hypnotics when given a renewable prescription during a brief episode of insomnia. Chronic heavy users of CNS depressants, including alcohol, show EEG patterns of decreased delta and REM sleep, increases in stage 1 and stage 2 sleep, frequent intermixing of EEG patterns from different stages of sleep, and loss of the normal pattern of REM-NREM cycling.

Sleep-disturbing CNS stimulants can include weight-reducing agents, caffeine, and stimulant drugs given for a mistaken diagnosis of narcolepsy. The ASDC reports that most people who habitually use stimulants originally had the drug prescribed for a medical condition. Sometimes insomniacs will take stimulants to relieve their daytime fatigue. They may also use hypnotics at night, thereby setting up a dangerous drug cycle. Use of stimulants leads to delayed sleep onset, a decline in total sleep time, reduction of delta and REM sleep, and frequent sleep interruptions. Treatment of DIMS that results from drug and alcohol use will include the stabilization of drug intake, gradual withdrawal from it, and therapy for any underlying sleep disturbance or psychopathology that may have led to the drug use. Often the original sleep problem will disappear once withdrawal from chronic hypnotics use is accomplished. More detail on withdrawal from hypnotics can be found in chapter 6.

DIMS Associated with Sleep-Induced Respiratory Impairment

Some individuals who breathe completely normally during the day experience serious and even life-threatening respiratory difficulties during sleep. Breathing may become excessively shallow during sleep or stop altogether as many as 500 times per night for periods lasting 10 to 120 seconds each. EEG recordings will show evidence of numerous partial or complete arousals from sleep during these periods. The most frequent kind of sleep-induced respiratory impairment is sleep apnea, of which there are 3 types. Central apnea most often has its source in the brainstem, leading to interference with the messages sent to the diaphragm. There is a cessation of airflow because the diaphragm does not attempt to move. Obstructive sleep apnea refers to a condition where the muscles of the upper airway relax during sleep, shrinking the airway, and causing breathing to become labored. The person continues to try to breathe, and may appear to be struggling to breathe, but is unable to do so. Mixed apneas start out as a central apnea followed by a phase of obstructive apnea.

It is rare for victims of sleep apnea to be aware of any of their nighttime respiratory difficulties. This points out the importance of obtaining a report from a bedpartner. For obstructive sleep apnea, probably the single most revealing symptom is the presence of loud snoring, often punctuated with a periodic gasping for breath. This kind of snoring is usually unaffected by changes in sleep position. Other signals of sleep apnea are obesity, a short, thick neck, serious morning headaches, and morning confusion. Medical evaluations occasionally reveal cardiac complications that are usually progressive unless the condition is reversed. Lack of oxygen during the night can cause a severe strain on an already dysfunctional cardiac system, possibly potentiating cardiac arrest. Physicians believe that sleep apnea may be the culprit when a seemingly healthy person mysteriously dies during sleep. The diagnosis of sleep apnea is made about 30 times more often in men than in women and appears to be more frequent in the elderly.

Sleep apnea may result in DIMS or in Disorders of Excessive Somnolence (DOES). A minority of individuals with sleep apnea will complain of difficulty maintaining sleep. In this case, the sleep problems are almost always associated with central or mixed apnea episodes that result in complete awakenings during the night. Much more often, a client will be unaware of the multiple arousals during the night and instead will complain of tremendous daytime sleepiness and of episodes of falling asleep during the day. The person is suffering from serious sleep deprivation. In the latter case, the most likely diagnosis is DOES associated with sleep-induced respiratory impairment.

The treatment of sleep apnea can range across a wide gamut of alternatives from simple to drastic. Mild cases can be relieved simply by sleeping in a sitting position. Moderate remedies include weight loss, removal of swollen adenoids, or use of a tongue-retaining device. More serious tactics are plastic surgery to move the jaw forward and to reposition the tongue, or a tracheostomy that is plugged during the day but unplugged at night to allow unobstructed ventilation. Under no circumstances should the apnea patient be given hypnotics, because these drugs are known to depress respiration, which could seriously aggravate the apnea problem (Hauri, 1982).

DIMS Associated with Nocturnal Myoclonus and "Restless Legs"

Nocturnal myoclonus refers to the occurrence during sleep of periodic episodes of repetitive and highly stereotyped jerking movements of the leg muscles. These movements do not occur during wakefulness, and the person is usually unaware of their occurrence at night. The contractions last up to 10 seconds with a remarkably regular interval of 20 to 40 seconds between jerks. The movements consist of extension of the big toe in combination with flexing of the ankle, knee, and sometimes the hip. Often an episode of myoclonus is followed by a partial arousal with a return to normal sleep between episodes. An individual can experience as many as 300 to 1000 myoclonic jerks in one night. Related behaviors that signal this disorder are leg cramps, family history of sleep maintenance disorders, restless sleep with disruption of the bed sheets, and falling out of bed. This disorder is usually seen in middle-aged and older individuals of both sexes. Some sleep experts believe that stress and emotional problems can cause the myclonus to appear or to worsen.

Restless legs syndrome occurs when the person is awake but the experience is so unpleasant that it frequently prevents the person from going to sleep. The chief symptom is an extremely uncomfortable, nervous or creeping sensation inside the legs while the person is sitting or lying down. The sensations cause an almost irresistible urge to move the legs or to walk about vigorously. Almost all people who suffer from restless legs also have nocturnal myoclonus although only a minority of myoclonus sufferers also experience restless legs. This syndrome becomes more severe with age, sleep deprivation, and pregnancy. About 30% of those afflicted have a family history of the syndrome.

As with sleep apnea, if the client complains of frequent nocturnal awakenings and unrefreshing sleep, the nocturnal myoclonus and restless legs are DIMS problems; if the complaint is of excessive daytime sleepiness, it is in the DOES category. Again, the report from a bedpartner in the case of intermittent and rhythmic leg kicking, may be crucial to this diagnosis. It is important not to confuse myoclonus with hypnic jerks, which are usually single body twitches or "startles" experienced at the beginning of sleep. The etiologies of both nocturnal myoclonus and restless legs are currently unexplained. The only known treatments for these two syndromes are medications. Treatment for restless legs has been much less successful than for myoclonus (Walsh et al., 1986.

DIMS Associated with Other Medical, Toxic, and Environmental Conditions

There are many other conditions that are known to disturb sleep: the pain of arthritis, CNS disorders, metabolic diseases, toxic effects from such substances as metals and drugs, and environmental conditions such as excessive noise or cold and disruptions from a bedpartner. Once the causative agent has been eliminated or reduced, the sleep problem usually improves.

Childhood-Onset DIMS

This particular subtype of DIMS appears to be rare. It consists of a persistent but unexplained history of insomnia that dates to at least well before puberty. Hauri and Olmstead (1980) report in their sleep laboratory studies that childhood-onset insomniacs, when compared with adult-onset insomniacs, took significantly longer to fall asleep, slept less, and showed excessive amounts of ill-defined REM sleep. They also demonstrated more soft neurological signs, such as hyper-kinesis, dyslexia, or attention-deficit disorders. The researchers specu-late that these individuals may suffer from a type of neurological impair-ment in the sleep-wake system that results in a pattern similar to persistent psychophysiological DIMS but with a more severe imbalance in the sleep-wake system. As a result, most of these individuals have insomnia from birth and do not require stress to trigger it. Hauri (1982) finds that many of these childhood-onset insomniacs are extremely sensitive to noise and to the effects of stimulants. Even one cup of tea ingested several hours before bedtime can seriously affect sleep. As for treatment of this type of poor sleeper, he reports success using low doses of Elavil.

DIMS Associated with Other Conditions

This category of sleep disturbance involves a number of conditions that can only be identified by polysomnography. One example shows atypical polysomnographic features, such as the mixing of EEG waves from different sleep stages, for instance when alpha or waking waves intrude into NREM sleep, resulting in nonrestorative sleep.

No DIMS Abnormality

Some people who complain of insomnia do not demonstrate any verifiable polysomnographic evidence of disturbed sleep. One example would be the naturally short sleeper who needs little sleep. The most common example, however, is the "subjective" insomniac. An apparently normal person makes a convincing and sincere report of fatigue from inadequate sleep but no objective evidence of a sleep problem can be found. In the past, this individual was given the pejorative label *pseudoinsomniac*, thus calling the person's character into question. However, current thinking is that the person is not a malingerer but may have a sleep disorder that is not yet known or that cannot be detected by available technology.

The report of subjective insomnia may involve perceptual or cognitive distortions that cannot be detected by polysomnography (Bootzin & Engle-Friedman, 1981). Currently accepted EEG criteria for the presence of sleep may not be sensitive enough to identify the subjective insomniac. During the early stages of sleep, subjective insomniacs may have stage reversals (e.g., intermingling of alpha and delta activity) or they may be sleeping so lightly that they perceive themselves to be awake still (Hauri & Olmstead, 1983). Haynes, Adams, West, Kamens, and Safranek (1982) suggest that these discrepancies between subjective and objective reports of sleep result because people differ in the physiological or cognitive markers on which they base their sleep onset estimates. Different individuals may not perceive the occurrence of sleep until they have reached stage 2 or stage 3. There is recent evidence that these subjective poor sleepers may show daytime impairment in spite of the absence of EEG patterns of disturbed sleep (Sugerman, Stern, & Walsh, 1985).

Because this category of DIMS is not well understood, it is difficult to make treatment recommendations. How many subjective insomniacs have actually been included in behavioral therapy studies is unknown. A sleep laboratory evaluation is required to make the diagnosis of subjective insomnia and most behavioral outcome studies have not been done in sleep laboratories. Also unknown is whether those who suffer from subjective and psychophysiological DIMS differ in their response to this kind of intervention. Because few participants in behavior therapy for insomnia are harmed by this experience, it is acceptable for the time being to treat these individuals with behavior therapy.

DISORDERS OF EXCESSIVE SOMNOLENCE (DOES)

Individuals need the amount of sleep that will permit them to be wide awake, alert, and energetic throughout the day. Some people, however, find that they are so sleepy during the day that they fall asleep inadvertently, even at times when they are active or when few other people fall asleep. The overly sleepy person may also experience microsleeps, or brief, hardly noticeable lapses. This kind of reaction can make a sleepy person accident prone and perhaps even dangerous when driving, flying, or operating machinery. Individuals who find themselves sleepy during the day to the point of falling asleep easily either have a problem that is preventing them from getting adequate nighttime sleep or they suffer from a pathological condition that leads to sleepiness all the time (Dement, 1983).

Although there are far more cases of DIMS in the population than of DOES, the latter make up a larger proportion of cases seen in sleep disorders centers. Because many of the DOES subtypes are serious and life-threatening and at the same time require complicated polysomnography to diagnose, individuals who complain of excessive daytime sleepiness should be referred to a sleep disorders center. DOES are more often associated with physiological and medical dysfunctions, many of which once diagnosed can be treated medically.

One of the primary techniques for objectively measuring whether sleepiness has reached pathological levels is the Multiple Sleep Latency Test. Individuals are given 4 to 6 opportunities during the day to take a nap in the sleep laboratory while hooked up for polysomnography. Those who complain of excessive daytime sleepiness will fall asleep rapidly (averaging less than 5 minutes) at each of these opportunities no matter what time of day it is. Rested good sleepers take 12 to 15 minutes or more to fall asleep or do not fall asleep when given the chance to take a daytime nap. Clients may also be asked to make 7-point ratings throughout the day of their level of alertness on the Stanford Sleepiness Scale.

There are multiple causes of DOES, some of which are the same as were found under the DIMS category. The subtypes that apply for both DIMS and DOES are those associated with psychophysiological factors, psychiatric disorders, use of drugs and alcohol, sleep-induced respiratory impairment, nocturnal myoclonus and restless legs, other medical, toxic, and environmental conditions, as well as no objective sleep abnormality. The important discriminating factor will be whether the chief complaint is of *disturbed sleep* or of *excessive daytime sleepiness.* Three subtypes are unique to DOES: idiopathic CNS hypersomnolence, DOES associated with other DOES syndromes, and narcolepsy.

The following comments on narcolepsy draw heavily upon the description provided by William Orr in Hauri (1982). Narcolepsy is a serious disorder that is marked by abnormal REM patterns, cataplexy, sleep paralysis, and hypnagogic hallucinations. In the sleep laboratory the narcoleptic shows early REM periods within the first 15 minutes of sleep. Cataplexy is a brief, sudden loss of skeletal muscle tone that is often observed after the person has had an emotional reaction such as laughter, anger, or excitement. The narcoleptic remains aware of the surroundings during the attack, which differentiates the event from a seizure. About 60% of narcoleptics experience cataplexy. Sleep paralysis is the total inability to move the muscles during the period of falling asleep or waking up. Though some normal individuals may experience this phenomenon while waking up, sleep paralysis at time of sleep onset is much more indicative of narcolepsy. Hypnagogic hallucinations are vivid dreamlike experiences that occur at the time of sleep onset.

Generally narcoleptics will begin to have periods of excessive daytime sleepiness in their early teens or twenties. Family history is a significant contributor, with males and females equally affected. This disorder is probably best conceptualized as an imbalance between the waking, REM, and NREM systems that can be experienced as anything from a slight nuisance to a severely incapacitating disease. Dement (1983) reports that in a series of narcoleptic patients, sleepiness resulted in occupational disability for 41%, 89% reported deteriorating relationships, and 91% had had accidents that they attributed to their sleepiness. Spouses, friends, and employers are likely to interpret the narcoleptic's frequent naps and sleepiness as lethargy, sloth, and lack of motivation.

DISORDERS OF THE SLEEP-WAKE SCHEDULE

Although insomnia and excessive daytime sleepiness have long been recognized by the medical community, scientists have only recently discovered that the sleep-wake rhythm itself can become disrupted. This diagnostic category may be mistaken for insomnia because some people who are suffering from the inability to sleep during conventional nighttime hours have no difficulty sleeping if allowed to do so at other times in the 24-hour cycle. They are suffering from delayed sleep phase syndrome. There is an apparent mismatch between their own personal circadian rhythm and society's timetable, the latter being oriented to the cycle of the earth's rotation about the sun. These individuals can be treated with a technique called chronotherapy, in which they are asked to delay their bedtime progressively by 2 to 3 hours each night. Eventually their bedtime will coincide with socially acceptable hours. Another category of disturbed circadian rhythm is the non-24-hour sleep-wake schedule where a person has a longer than 24-hour cycle, such as 26 or 28 hours. By getting up at the same time each morning (usually imposed by job expectations) and then going to bed later each night because they are not yet sleepy, these people eventually become seriously sleep-deprived.

A more temporary version of sleep-wake schedule difficulties is brought on by sudden work shift changes and also by jet lag from crossing many time zones in a short period. In the latter case, a person's biological rhythms lag behind the time shown on the local clock. Temporary sleep problems may develop if a person is forced to work a different shift, one that occurs during one's regular sleeping time. However, irregular schedules of frequently shifting sleep and wake time can lead to a chronic sleep problem from a disturbance of the circadian rhythm. Those who are younger and good sleepers are evidently less vulnerable to the effects of jet lag or of work-shift changes than are older persons and poor sleepers.

PARASOMNIAS

The term *parasomnia* refers to disorders associated with sleep, sleep stages, or partial arousals. Parasomnias are undesirable experiences that occur either exclusively during sleep or are aggravated by sleep. Examples of parasomnias include sleepwalking, sleep terrors, enuresis, dream anxiety attacks, bruxism, sleep-related gastroesophageal reflux, and sleep-related cluster headaches. It has been estimated that 5% of the population of the United States suffers from one of these parasomnias (Hauri, 1982). Some of these disorders are found mainly in children (e.g., sleepwalking, sleep terrors, enuresis) and tend to disappear in adolescence or adulthood. Treatments for the others are specific to the individual symptoms and include behavior therapy as well as strictly medical approaches.

PREVALENCE AND TREATMENT OF SLEEP DISORDERS

There are many estimates of the number of people in the population who suffer from disturbance of their sleep. A number of wide-scale surveys have been done that document sleep disturbance as a widespread problem in the United States. However, in these surveys, "insomnia" or "sleep disturbance" is by necessity defined globally. Therefore, there are no definitive figures for the prevalence of all the ASDC sleep disorders within the general population. Most reports of this nature have to do with the numbers of the various types of sleep problems that have been seen in sleep disorders centers. These figures are not representative of a broader population because they are heavily weighted toward the most serious kinds of sleep disturbances.

Coleman et al. (1982) published prevalence figures from a national survey of 3900 patients over 2 years at 11 sleep disorders centers. Each patient was evaluated through polysomnography and given an ASDC diagnosis. For the four major ASDC categories the percentage diagnosed were: DIMS (31%), DOES (51%), sleep-wake schedule disorders (3%), and parasomnias (15%). Within the DIMS category, 15% were diagnosed as psychophysiological DIMS, 35% had DIMS with psychiatric disturbance, 12% as having DIMS associated with the use of drugs and alcohol, 6% with apnea, 12% with nocturnal myoclonus or restless legs, 9% had subjective insomnia, and 12% were diagnosed in the remaining three subtypes. Within DOES, 43% were diagnosed as having sleep apnea and 25% as having narcolepsy. Each of the other subcategories appeared in small percentages including nocturnal myoclonus and restless legs (4%).

How does a practitioner decide if a client complaining of sleep disturbance should be evaluated in a sleep disorders center? These evaluations are very expensive and not all communities have this kind of facility. Are there some clients with whom you might try a course of behavior therapy before opting for the more extensive evaluation? If the person is not elderly, if the primary complaint is sleep onset insomnia, and if, using questionnaires and interviews, you can rule out any evidence of sleep apnea, nocturnal myoclonus, restless legs, or narcolepsy, then you are probably safe in not recommending an initial evaluation using polysomnography. Because excessive daytime sleepiness is so often associated with serious organic sleep pathology, anyone with this complaint should have a sleep laboratory evaluation. What to do with the person with chronic, unremitting sleep maintenance insomnia is more problematic. This person may be suffering from objective or subjective DIMS, in which case behavior therapy would be appropriate. However, the client might also be suffering from one of the organic sleep disorders that disrupts the maintenance of sleep, such as sleep apnea or nocturnal myoclonus. If interview or history data, including information from a bedpartner, reveal no evidence of organic sleep disorder, it may be acceptable to try a brief course of behavior therapy. However, if the client does not respond to the treatment, he or she should probably be referred for the more extensive evaluation that only a sleep disorders center can provide.

It is clear that many sleep disturbances are based upon underlying psychiatric, medical, or environmental factors. Treatment of these cases should always begin with the removal of the primary or initial cause of the disorder. However, if the poor sleeper has had insomnia for more than a few months, it is likely that secondary psychological factors, such as learned maladaptive bedtime behaviors or the development of performance anxiety, are contributing to the sleeping problem. Exacerbation cycles can develop when the client becomes obsessed with the loss of sleep and with the task of getting more sleep. Relationships and job performance may be compromised. In such cases, it is likely that the person needs a behavioral intervention in addition to psychiatric or medical treatment.

Chapter 4
Behavioral Treatment of Insomnia

Over the past 20 years a number of theoretical perspectives have been used to explain persistent insomnia. At least five competing psychological theories have guided thinking and treatment planning: (a) somatic arousal, (b) emotional arousal, (c) performance anxiety, (d) stimulus control, and (e) cognitive arousal. Of these, somatic arousal, stimulus control, and cognitive arousal have been most influential in the stimulation of treatment outcome research. Proponents of each of the dominant theories of the development of insomnia recommend particular interventions that fit their own viewpoint. In this chapter, the reader will find a brief overview of the most prominent causative theories of and treatment approaches to persistent insomnia.

SOMATIC AROUSAL

The first theory to have a significant impact on the planning of behavior therapies for chronic insomnia was that of somatic arousal. Advocates of this point of view believe that individuals with poor sleep have heightened physiological arousal and muscle tension that is antagonistic to sleep. Presumably, this tension builds up gradually during the day because the individual has no effective mechanism to expend it. The somatic arousal hypothesis gained initial support from Monroe's 1967 comparison of good and poor laboratory sleepers. Monroe found that just prior to and during sleep, poor sleepers in contrast to good sleepers had elevated levels of autonomic activity on a number of measures such as temperature and heart rate. Subsequent physiological studies, however, have not produced convincing evidence that a heightened state of presleep somatic arousal is a major causative factor in insomnia (VanOot, Lane, & Borkovec, 1984). Furthermore, treatment outcome studies have generally not found a relationship between any decline in physiological activity achieved during relaxation training and either subjective or objective measures of sleep. Lichstein and Rosenthal (1980) found that in a sample of 296 insomniacs, only 5% claimed that somatic arousal alone described their presleep state.

Hauri (1979) has posed the possibility that autonomic arousal may not necessarily be the cause of sleep disturbance, but instead is the byproduct of sleeplessness. He reports that a number of researchers have found signs of autonomic arousal in healthy volunteers after experimentally induced sleep deprivation. Some poor sleepers may develop autonomic arousal after a period of consistently disturbed sleep. If somatic arousal does play a role in the development and maintenance of persistent insomnia, its contribution may be limited to particular subtypes of this sleep disturbance.

For centuries, people have believed that physical tension blocks the onset of sleep. Many of the popular remedies for poor sleep are designed to get a person to relax before bedtime. Some examples are drinking a glass of wine or a cup of tea, taking a warm bath, listening to music or a recording of the surf, or taking a walk. Even though there has not been strong research corroboration of a physiological arousal basis of insomnia, a large number of studies have been fostered by that original 1967 Monroe research. In particular, there have been many treatment outcome investigations of methods designed to alleviate such somatic tension. Many behavior therapists subscribe to the philosophy that if poor sleepers can learn to relax at bedtime, they will have less difficulty falling asleep. An added benefit of this therapeutic approach is that relaxation training may enable the individual to cope more adequately with the everyday stresses that might lead to sleeping problems in the first place.

Anxiety-reduction strategies that have been applied to insomnia include: progressive relaxation, autogenic training, transcendental meditation, biofeedback, and hypnosis. Of these, progressive relaxation has been the most thoroughly subjected to scientific scrutiny. Although there are variations among practitioners, Bernstein and Borkovec (1973) have described one relaxation approach for use with poor sleepers. When progressive relaxation techniques are used, clients are usually asked to practice the new skills twice a day, for about 20 minutes, with the last practice occurring upon retiring.

In addition to tension reduction through muscle relaxation, this state of low physiological arousal can also be achieved by a cognitive relaxation strategy called autogenic training (Schultz & Luthe, 1959). Imagery and self-suggestion are used to influence various physiological processes. Another somewhat related method for achieving a state of relaxation is through the systematic and daily practice of clinically standardized transcendental meditation (Carrington, 1977). This technique involves two daily sessions during which the client silently focuses attention upon a *mantra*, which is an undifferentiated and repetitive sound thought to have soothing properties.

Relaxation can also be induced through biofeedback. Most insomnia researchers have been interested in frontalis electromyograph (EMG) biofeedback in the belief that frontalis muscle relaxation will generalize to other muscle groups, resulting in a global relaxation effect. Another modality of biofeedback used in the remediation of sleeping problems is sensory motor rhythm (SMR) biofeedback. The latter is not designed to promote reduced muscle tension but is instead supposed to strengthen certain components of the sleep circuitry (e.g., the enhancement of sleep spindling rhythms). Biofeedback sessions usually last from 30 to 45 minutes with the number of sessions required to reach criterion varying widely; for example, in Hauri's sleep laboratory the range of sessions was 15 to 60 (Hauri, 1981).

EMOTIONAL AROUSAL

Some investigators believe that the arousal attributed to the insomniac is an emotional arousal that results from an anxious perfectionistic personality style. Frequently, the insomniac is a person prone both to internalizing reactions to stressful life events and to somatizing unresolved conflicts. These inadequate coping responses lead to a heightened emotional state and concomitant physiological arousal. In addition to having fewer adaptive coping mechanisms for stress, there is some evidence that the poor sleeper may undergo increased life stress during the year in which the sleep disturbance first appears (Healy et al., 1981). Proponents of this causative theory would also advocate anxiety-reducing strategies as well as training in stress management and cognitive restructuring.

Although the most frequently used measure has been the Minnesota Multiphasic Personality Inventory (MMPI), a wide array of other personality tests has also been given to poor sleepers. The results of these studies have been surprisingly consistent. In contrast to those who have no problems with sleep, insomniacs demonstrate more psychopathology. For example, Levin, Bertelson, and Lacks (1984) found that 53% of their insomniac MMPI profiles had at least one clinical scale with a T-score equal to or above 70 compared with a group of good sleepers in which only 16% had elevated MMPI scores. In general, however, insomniac MMPI scores were not highly elevated. Across 9 MMPI clinical scales (excluding Mf), mild insomniacs had a mean scale score of 57.9, severe insomniacs of 60.0, and good sleepers of

53.0. Personality test research with insomnia sufferers shows a clinical picture of an introverted, worried, and inhibited individual who is mildly depressed (Borkovec, 1982; Youkilis & Bootzin, 1981). "In essence, such a pattern reflects significantly more pathology, neuroticism, social withdrawal, somatic symptoms, and unhappiness" (Beutler, Thornby, & Karacan, 1978, p. 67). The same pattern emerges across many samples and does not seem related to chronicity or severity of the insomnia.

Again, we must also consider the chicken-versus-the-egg question. Sleep disturbance over some length of time appears to decrease a person's sense of general competence or confidence in the ability to handle problems. This negative self-attitude may then help to usher in feelings of depression that only exacerbate the sleep problem and lead to a downward spiral of lessening sleep and lowering mood. Sleep deprivation, like any stress, can precipitate any predisposition to psychopathology. If depression, somatic arousal, and psychopathology are the results of disrupted sleep, they should abate with sleep improvement. If they are etiological aspects of insomnia, these factors should remain unchanged with sleep improvement (Hauri, 1979). In Hauri's laboratory, of 30 insomnia sufferers treated with various forms of biofeedback, 12 showed EEG-verified improvement. A year after treatment, these 12 had significantly lowered depression and hostility, but not anxiety. Hauri interprets these findings to mean that depression and hostility were the consequences of the poor sleep but anxiety was probably more of an etiological factor. Both those subjects who were treated but did not show improvement and control subjects who were not treated generally showed a worsening of all three factors.

PERFORMANCE ANXIETY AND LOW SELF-EFFICACY

Many individuals who complain of poor sleep also suffer anxiety and low self-concept that are specific to their sleep disturbance. It is not unusual to find very high performance anxiety and low sense of self-efficacy among those who suffer from persistent insomnia. In fact, these two elements may become primary in maintaining the sleep disorder. As a person first begins to experience difficulty with sleep, he or she is likely to attempt to control the sleep process voluntarily; in other words to *try harder* to fall asleep. These attempts to hasten sleep onset may have the opposite effect of that intended by evoking an increase in autonomic arousal that actually delays the onset of sleep. This urgency to fall asleep is probably related to the anxious, perfectionistic personality style — always wanting to be at one's best and not wanting lack of sleep to interfere with the next day's work. The stage is set for the vicious cycle of performance anxiety. Trying harder to fall asleep leads to anxiety and tension that impede sleep and this situation leads to trying even harder, and so on (Ascher, 1980). The effect of a strong conscious effort to fall asleep has been experimentally demonstrated with good sleepers by asking them to fall asleep as fast as possible with a cash prize for the most successful attempt. Baseline time to fall asleep in a sleep laboratory for the experimental group was 11.6 minutes. On the night of the experimentally induced motivation, these subjects took 21.9 minutes to fall asleep (Shaffer, Dickel, Marik, & Slak, 1985).

Most poor sleepers do not experience sleep difficulties every night. Even those with the most severe insomnia have one or two nights in a typical week during which they will sleep adequately. But they never know which nights those will be. This night-to-night variability of sleep can lead the poor sleeper to feel impotent and to conclude that sleep is uncontrollable. Yet the majority of people sleep well most of the time with little apparent difficulty. This fact can lead the insomnia sufferer to doubt his or her personal stability and level of competence not only to sleep but to accomplish other life tasks as well. These uncertainties again add to the level of tension and to the insomnia exacerbation cycle (Killen & Coates, 1979). Ironically, therapy designed to help the performance-anxious client get better sleep may actually exacerbate the problem by promoting additional effort and focus on sleep.

Many people who experience poor sleep have been told by family and friends not to try so hard. As it turns out, though the advice is simple, it may make very good sense. Trying harder to fall asleep may only increase the anxiety. Probably one of the most unique and creative treatments to be used for persistent insomnia has been paradoxical intention. Ascher (1980) reasoned that performance anxiety over sleep might be reduced if clients were encouraged to focus upon trying *not* to fall asleep. Clients would presumably worry less about something that they were not trying to accomplish. These researchers gave insomniacs the paradoxical instructions to try to stay awake the entire night, not to allow themselves to fall asleep. Some individuals given these directions were unable to complete them and instead fell asleep. Additional details about the use of paradoxical intention as a treatment for insomnia can be found in Ascher (1980).

STIMULUS CONTROL

For many of us, much of what we do is influenced by the time, place, and circumstances in which we find ourselves. The sitmuli or characteristics of a situation become paired with the behavior that occurs in that situation. The characteristics of the situation then become a signal or cue for that behavior. Some familiar examples are: wanting popcorn the minute you step into a movie theater lobby even if you have just finished a large meal; being hungry to eat lunch because the clock indicates noon; craving a cigarette each time you drink a cup of coffee; experiencing anxiety when the phone rings in the middle of the night but not when it rings during the day. For most individuals the bed and bedroom have a long association with the rapid onset of sleepiness and so serve as cues to feel drowsy and fall asleep without delay. A certain set of prebedtime routines, a favorite pillow, and a particular position in bed are examples of some of the cues that promote the onset of sleep. These cues become so strong that a good sleeper may go to bed with every intention of watching a television show or reading for a while and within minutes is struggling to stay awake.

Yet for many poor sleepers, the bed and bedroom are not cues for drowsiness and the onset of sleep. Instead, these places have become strong signals or discriminative stimuli for alertness and sleeplessness. According to Bootzin (1977), an operant conditioning factor is at work here. Difficulty in falling asleep is the result of inadequate stimulus control. The bed and bedroom and even thoughts about going to bed have been associated with sleep-incompatible behaviors long enough so that they elicit an aroused rather than a drowsy state. Bootzin hypothesizes that chronic insomniacs use the bed for many of the activities of living: eating, talking on the phone, watching television, studying, and others. Perhaps the most important sleep-incompatible behaviors engaged in by the poor sleeper are worrying, problem solving, and planning in bed. The most significant worry is likely to become that of not being able to sleep, with all its attendant frustration and anxiety.

The connection between the bed and lack of sleep becomes so strong in some insomnia sufferers that the bed and bedroom become potent aversive stimuli as well. I have had clients tell me that their bed is the "enemy" and that they dread having to go to bed because of the attached associations. Interestingly, this connection usually exists only with their own bed and not with other sleeping places. Many of these people have no trouble sleeping in a chair in front of the television or in a hotel or even in a sleep laboratory! In contrast, good sleepers often have difficulty sleeping outside of their familiar bed site.

This type of conditioning may be the original cause of the sleep difficulties or it may take place after normal sleep has been disrupted by some other cause, such as stress or illness. In the latter case, the conditioned arousal at bedtime maintains the insomnia once the original stress abates. Those who ascribe to this operant analysis of insomnia approach the alleviation of sleep difficulties from a very different direction. The treatment for insomnia that has been derived from this conditioning theory is called stimulus control. It was developed in 1972 by Richard Bootzin at Northwestern University (Bootzin, 1972). Other researchers refer to similar approaches, such as lifestyle management (Lichstein and Fischer, 1985) or habit restructuring (Turner & DiTomasso, 1980). All focus on environmental factors and daily living routines that are thought to influence sleep.

The chief feature of Bootzin's method consists of teaching people to reassociate the bed and bedroom with rapid sleep onset by curtailing all sleep-incompatible behaviors in the bedroom that serve as cues for staying awake. Examples of such activities are eating, arguing, writing, watching television, talking on the phone, planning tomorrow's schedule, or simply lying awake. To prevent the association between the bed and the behavior of lying awake, clients are instructed to go to bed only when drowsy, to get out of bed any time a waking period of 10 minutes has passed, and not to return to bed until sleepy again. This sequence is repeated as many times as necessary throughout the night.

Although it does not really fit with an operant paradigm, the establishment of a regular sleep schedule is also included in Bootzin's stimulus control methods. The development of a consistent sleep rhythm is facilitated by requiring a regular awakening time each day and by the elimination of naps. Eventually, people who follow these guidelines will become drowsy at approximately the same time each night. This set of stimulus control rules forms the core of a widely used behavior therapy for persistent insomnia. The strong research support for it will be outlined later in this chapter. Stimulus control therapy also is the primary approach advocated in this practitioner guidebook. It will be described in detail in chapters 6, 7, and 8.

COGNITIVE AROUSAL

Because there has been little experimental support for the hypothesis that physiological arousal causes insomnia, behaviorists have recently turned their attention to cognitive arousal. There is much more evidence that cognitive arousal plays an important role in the etiology and maintenance of sleep difficulties. One of the chief complaints of poor sleepers is that they are unable to control their cognitions while lying in bed at night. That is, they complain of "racing thoughts."

Lichstein and Rosenthal (1980) surveyed 296 insomniacs who had a mean duration of 11 years of sleep complaints and a mean latency to sleep of 89 minutes. Two possible causes of insomnia were explained to these subjects. One factor was described as somatic arousal at bedtime with such examples as feeling restless, tossing, and a sweating body. The other causative factor was cognitive arousal described as an active mind at bedtime, worrying, planning, and difficulty controlling thoughts. Participants were asked to decide if they thought that their sleep difficulties were attributable to somatic arousal, cognitive arousal, both types of arousal, or neither of these factors. Only 5% of these poor sleepers claimed that somatic arousal alone described their presleep state. Another 35% claimed that their insomnia was caused by both somatic and cognitive arousal. Five percent endorsed neither of these forms of arousal. The largest number of subjects (55%) perceived cognitive arousal to be the cause of their sleep problems. This means that a total of 90% implicated cognitive arousal in their insomnia. Of those who believed both cognitive and somatic arousal contributed to their insomnia, cognitive arousal was considered to be the most disruptive to sleep.

Nicassio, Mendlowitz, Fussell, and Petras (1985) found that responses on both the somatic arousal and the cognitive arousal subscales of their Pre-Sleep Arousal Scale differentiated poor sleepers from good sleepers; however, the cognitive subscale was more strongly associated with measures of sleep difficulty. For example, correlation between time to fall asleep and the somatic subscale was .29, but correlation between time to fall asleep and the cognitive subscale was .59. It appears that a large number of poor sleepers have a surplus of uncontrollable thoughts at bedtime that may arouse the autonomic nervous system and interfere with sleep. These thoughts also tend to be rated as more negative and worrisome than those of good sleepers (Borkovec, Lane, and VanOot, 1981). Poor sleepers complain of racing thoughts, general worries, and specific worries about being able to sleep (Borkovec, 1982).

Some researchers have been able to manipulate experimentally the effect of cognitive arousal upon sleep. For example, Gross and Borkovec (1982) conducted such a study with 38 good sleepers who had no fear of public speaking. The subjects were instructed during a daytime nap session to go to sleep as quickly as possible. They were randomly assigned to one of three instructional sets: (a) only to fall asleep; (b) to fall asleep and be asked to give a 3-minute speech upon awakening; and (c) to fall asleep and upon awakening be asked to give a 3-minute speech on a specific topic. Subjects in the third group, who knew they were to make a speech and who knew the topic of the speech, took significantly longer to fall asleep (54 minutes) than the first two groups (31 and 29 minutes, respectively), as verified by EEG. Interestingly, this cognitive intrusion effect occurred independently of any evidence of elevated physiological activity.

A second aspect of the role of cognition in insomnia revolves around the phenomenology of the poor sleeper during sleep. In the sleep laboratory, when good sleepers who are asleep by EEG criteria are awakened and questioned about their sleep, they almost always report having been asleep, while the majority of insomniacs (both ASDC objective and subjective subtypes) report that they were awake (e.g., Borkovec et al., 1981). By objective criteria, both groups were asleep; however, their subjective experience was quite different. Although both groups had achieved stage 2 sleep, the poor sleepers did show a greater variability in the number of stage reversals, whereas the transition from awake to asleep was much smoother for the good sleepers. This obsessively worrying presleep state is a much more active and stimulating activity than the more passive hypnagogic fantasy process that good sleepers usually report takes place in the presleep interval (Coursey, Buchsbaum, & Frankel, 1975). Something about the amount and/or kind of presleep cognitive activity in the insomniac appears to create a phenomenology during sleep that is much more like being awake than it is like being asleep.

A third area of support for the role of cognitive intrusion comes from the treatment outcome literature. In a number of investigations that have used cognitive control interventions, the level of cognitive arousal has been substantially reduced during treatment (e.g., Mitchell, 1979). This lowering of presleep intrusive cognitions has not been observed following treatment with progressive relaxation (e.g., Woolfolk & McNulty, 1983). Mitchell concludes that control of the racing thoughts and worries that plague insomnia sufferers is a particularly relevant treatment target for the sleep onset insomniac.

Probably the most well-known folk remedy for poor sleep is to lie in bed and count sheep. Without realizing it, individuals who engage in this activity are using a cognitive control technique. A good deal of current research interest surrounds this viewpoint and a number of treatment approaches have developed from it. Examples of specific interventions are cognitive refocusing, imagery, ocular relaxation, and meditation.

Cognitive refocusing involves training in a number of attention refocusing techniques including external focus, internal focus, and body sensation. The goal is to teach clients to concentrate on these strategies rather than on sleep-incompatible thoughts and worries. Additional details of these strategies are presented in chapter 9. A close kin to cognitive refocusing is transcendental meditation, in which attention is trained upon a particular word or mantra. Although meditation has already been described as a method of tension reduction, some researchers have conceptualized meditation as a facilitator of cognitive control (Schoicket, Bertelson, & Lacks, 1987). A similar cognitive control technique is guided imagery. In this procedure, individuals are guided through a particular visual scene by the therapist, who follows a written script. Clients close their eyes and focus all of their attention on the images being described. Some of these scenes are meant to distract (e.g., a lemon being sliced) and some have the added goal of promoting relaxation (e.g., a pleasant beach scene).

Ocular relaxation is a technique developed by E. Jacobson (1938) as part of his methods for progressive muscle relaxation. He used eye-movement exercises to induce "blank minds" in his subjects. These ocular procedures were dropped from progressive relaxation as practiced by most behavior therapists. However, Lichstein and his colleagues have pursued an interest in ocular relaxation as a treatment for insomnia. Like Jacobson, they consider reduction of ocular movement to suppress cognitive activity (Lichstein & Sallis, 1982). The procedure involves a systematic pattern of moving the eyes in different directions and holding the position for 7 seconds. In between movements, the subject focuses for 40 seconds on relaxing sensations in the eyes. Outcome reports of the utility of ocular relaxation in the treatment of insomnia have been mixed (Lichstein & Fischer, 1985).

Which of these five factors is the true cause of persistent insomnia? Each of these components may play the major role of precipitating and maintaining sleep disturbance in certain individuals who suffer from this disorder. The typical poor sleeper will likely be influenced by all or most of these elements. The scenario may run something like this. Many people experience temporary sleep disturbance during a period of some stressful life situation such as childbirth, loss of a job, or illness of some family member. A subset of these individuals will respond to this disruption of their sleep with worry about being able to sleep and about the next-day consequences of insufficient sleep. They tend to be the anxious and "worrying" kind anyway. Typically, persons from this group will then try harder to fall asleep. Each night as they continue to have trouble getting to sleep, they worry more about it and become progressively more anxious. The time they take to fall asleep lengthens and they begin to fret about other things: rehashing the day's events, listing what has to be accomplished the next day, rehearsing things to say to others, composing various lists and inventories, and so on. As time passes, these thoughts begin to pick up speed so that they can be described as "racing," and the budding insomniac feels lessening control over these thoughts. If asked in the middle of the night what he or she is thinking of, the insomniac might truthfully answer "everything" or "hundreds of things."

This experience of uncontrolled cognitive arousal is very unpleasant and may become associated with the bed and bedroom where the negative experience has so often begun to take place. The sleepless person may now begin to view the bed in very negative terms, and the bed may even become a cue for sleeplessness and racing thoughts. In an attempt to get more sleep this person begins to take naps, to go to bed before drowsy in order to get a head start on sleep, and to sleep later in the mornings to make up for lost sleep. Soon the sleep schedule becomes erratic and more energy goes into the quest for precious sleep. Activities and exercise may be curtailed because of excessive fatigue. After repeated experiences of failure, the person becomes more self-preoccupied and feels inadequate because such a simple and natural process as getting a good night's sleep eludes control. Life's regular challenges and stresses appear overwhelming. Mild depression may set in.

Due either to the anxiety or to the depression or both, the insomniac may become worn down and start to experience other health problems. Friction with a spouse, friends and co-workers, lowered efficiency at work, and more self-doubt and hopelessness may follow. In desperation, the insomniac may turn to sleep medications with their associated problems of tolerance, dependence, disrupted sleep architecture, and further erosion of daytime performance. The person's life becomes one large exacerbation cycle and downward spiral. By the time an insomniac reaches a behavior therapist, he or she will have spent an average of 14 years in this pattern and will now be taking 1 or 2 hours to fall asleep or will be awake for this amount of time in the middle of the night. The picture just described is one that will be familiar to most individuals who seek help for their sleep disturbance.

RESEARCH FINDINGS

There appear to be large numbers of sleep-disturbed individuals in our society for whom behavioral interventions are appropriate. This group of poor sleepers has been treated successfully with a variety of behavioral techniques that have developed from several theoretical orientations regarding the cause of insomnia. All of these techniques have had some measure of success as demonstrated by their consistent superiority over both no-treatment conditions and placebo conditions. However, none of these approaches has produced an entirely successful treatment for insomnia. In this section, a brief description of the research findings for 4 of these treatments will be provided. The 4 strategies covered are (a) progressive relaxation, (b) paradoxical intention, (c) stimulus control, and (d) cognitive control. For those readers who would like more details on these methods and others, a number of excellent reviews are available, such as Bootzin and Nicassio (1978), Borkovec (1982), Lichstein and Fischer (1985), and VanOot, Lane, and Borkovec (1984).

A number of general conclusions can be drawn from the literature. Although there has been good treatment success, benefits are best described as moderate. The majority of participants in therapy outcome studies have not become good sleepers. Lichstein and Fischer (1985) in a survey of 48 studies of 16 different treatments found that at baseline the average sleep onset latency (SOL) was 66 minutes, a figure that was reduced to 35 minutes at posttreatment. However, in contrast to results often observed in behavioral work with smokers and the obese, improved sleep following behavior therapy is very robust. Research has shown strong maintenance of treatment effects over as long a period as a year. In a sample of clients we have treated, 157 with sleep onset problems reduced their baseline SOL from 72 minutes to 40 minutes after treatment, 36 minutes at short-term follow-up, and 33 minutes at 1-year follow-up. The respective wake time after sleep onset (WASO) figures for 117 individuals with sleep maintenance complaints were 88, 54, 46, and 48 minutes. These results are more impressive when you keep in mind that persistent insomnia does not spontaneously remit; no treatment groups do not improve.

The most frequently researched behavioral approach to insomnia is progressive relaxation. Borkovec (1982) reports that there have been 4 outcome studies of this technique that employed the EEG as the dependent measure (e.g., Borkovec & Weerts, 1976) and 13 studies that relied upon self-report. Although the various relaxation procedures were effective, they did not generally produce dramatic reductions of sleep disturbance. Improvement from self-report averaged 45% and from EEG (stage 1) averaged 59%. Bootzin and Nicassio (1978), after surveying many studies, found that the average reduction of the target behavior as a result of relaxation training was less than 50%. Lichstein and Fischer (1985), summarizing 24 studies of progressive relaxation, found a 43% rate of improvement.

Paradoxical intention has been studied much less than have either progressive relaxation or stimulus control. The results have also been less consistent across studies. Borkovec (1982) found an average 58% improvement in self-report across 4 studies. Lichstein and Fischer (1985) found reductions of 46% in 9 studies. In our own work we found only an 18% improvement rate for this strategy (Lacks, Bertelson, Gans, & Kunkel, 1983). We also found that subjects who suffered from mild to moderate insomnia showed slight increases in sleep disturbance after being treated with paradoxical intention. In a report of 6 case studies, Espie and Lindsay (1985) found considerable variability in response to paradoxical intention with half the clients showing a rapid reduction in SOL and the other half showing exacerbation of their sleep problems. However, Turner and Ascher (1979) found good success rates for paradoxical intention, equivalent to that achieved with progressive relaxation and stimulus control.

The second most studied technique is stimulus control. As a rule, this form of behavior therapy has shown the highest rates of effectiveness in the treatment of insomnia. In his review, Borkovec (1982) reported overall self-report improvement rates of 70% and Lichstein and Fischer (1985) reported rates of 58% across 13 studies. Participants in these studies have come from a wide range of sources, ages, chronicity, and severity of their sleep problems. Furthermore, in studies in which stimulus control has been directly compared with other strategies it has generally shown the best results (e.g., Lacks, Bertelson, Gans, & Kunkel, 1983; Morin & Azrin, 1987). Although the success of this approach has not yet been documented with polysomnography, Morin, Duffee, Zande, and Azrin (1986) did corroborate reductions of sleep complaints on an electromechanical timer.

Few investigations have been conducted on the efficacy of cognitive control methods for alleviating insomnia. Morin and his colleagues in 2 separate studies found that a posttreatment stimulus control was more effective than imagery training in reducing the sleep maintenance complaints of adults (Morin & Azrin, 1987) and of older adults (Morin et al., 1986). However, two unpublished studies from our own research program have shown that a broader training program in cognitive refocusing was equal to stimulus control with cognitively aroused sleep onset insomniacs (T. W. Cook & Lacks, 1986) and that meditation produced about the same results with sleep maintenance insomniacs as did stimulus control (Schoicket et al., 1987). Furthermore, unlike other process variables, presleep cognitive intrusion has been the only factor to show reductions that parallel reductions in sleep disturbance (e.g., Woolfolk & McNulty, 1983). Clearly this technique is one that calls for further study.

Chapter 5
Diagnosis of Disorders of Initiating and Maintaining Sleep (Insomnia)

There is no specific disease that is called insomnia. Instead, insomnia is a complaint that can stem from a multitude of factors including organic pathology, painful medical conditions, physiological dysfunction, hypnotic medication or other drug use, psychopathology, emotional arousal and stress, personality style, and learned behaviors. Assessment of the nature of the sleep disturbance, the source of the complaint, and the consequences to each individual will be a complex task, but it is an essential one for optimal treatment planning. A complete assessment of a complaint of insomnia or sleep disturbance will include:

- Detailed personal history
- Psychological inventories
- Daily sleep diaries
- Objective sleep measures
- Specialized measures for insomnia
- Medical and sleep laboratory evaluation

Behavior therapy will only work well as the primary intervention for insomnia caused by certain conditions though it may be a useful adjunct treatment for insomnia from other factors. In some cases, behavior therapy may not be the treatment of choice at all. In arriving at a diagnosis for the sleep-disturbed individual, the clinician will need to utilize the information and materials in this chapter in conjunction with the background material that has been provided in the preceding chapters.

DETAILED PERSONAL HISTORY

Our research team has developed a three-tiered approach to obtaining a detailed personal history of sleep disturbance. The three specialized instruments are the Insomnia Phone Screening, the Sleep History Questionnaire, and the Structured Sleep History Interview. We always begin with the Insomnia Phone Screening Sheet (see Table 5.1), which is filled out during the initial telephone inquiry from the client. This form enables us to collect the desired information in a standard format and also reminds us of the questions that we want to be sure to ask. From this preliminary conversation with a prospective client, we try to determine if we have an appropriate treatment to offer or if the person should be referred to another source for help. Primary examples of

Table 5.1. Insomnia Treatment Phone Screening Sheet

Name _____ Date _____

Address _____

Phone and best contact times: Home _____Work _____

Age _____Education _____Referral source _____

Rank problems: Sleep onset _____Sleep maintenance _____Early awakening _____

Amount awake at night _____ Number of nights/week _____Chronicity_____

Sleep medications (including over-the-counter)_____

_____

Willing to give up sleep medication during treatment?   YES   NO

Ever use alcohol to aid sleep?   YES   NO

Explain_____

Other medications currently taken (reason, name, dosage, frequency)_____

_____

Who prescribed medications? _____

Insomnia related to physical complaints? (e.g., pain)   YES   NO

Explain _____

Current psychotherapy for insomnia?   YES   NO

Explain_____

Previous behavior therapy for insomnia?   YES   NO

Explain_____

****

Disposition

_____ Accepted for in-person screening.   Date and time _____

_____ Recontact.   Reason _____

_____ Client undecided, will call us.

_____ Not suitable.   Reason _____

individuals whom we refer elsewhere are those who appear to have organic sleep pathology, those with some serious psychiatric disorder such as schizophrenia, bipolar affective disorder, current major depressive episode, or substance abuse, and those who have some serious, painful medical condition (e.g., arthritis) that disrupts sleep. If any question on this screening form is answered positively we then pursue it further to see if the caller falls into one of these broad categories for which behavior therapy for insomnia has not yet been shown to be applicable. For example, a person who uses alcohol to promote sleep may upon additional questioning turn out to have a serious problem with alcohol dependence. When asked about current medications, some applicants will reveal that they take antipsychotic or antidepressant medication for serious psychopathology.

At the time of the initial phone inquiry, we also explain briefly the procedures and cost of the therapy. The intervention is described as a nondrug behavioral treatment for insomnia that involves learning new sleep habits and practices. Participants meet once a week for 4 weeks in small groups in sessions that last 60 to 90 minutes. If the caller is still interested we then schedule an in-person assessment session that lasts from 2 to 3 hours.

In the next phase there are a number of choices. The evaluator can have the client fill out the Sleep History Questionnaire (see Table 5.2) and then follow up those responses listed in Table 5.3 by administering selected parts of the Structured Sleep History Interview (see Table 5.4); or the questionnaire may be eliminated altogether and the entire structured interview given. Of course, the latter approach will be more time consuming but it is also more thorough. These two instruments have items that are organized into 7 broad categories; the item numbers for each of the 2 instruments coincide up through item number 34, after which 5 additional items are inserted into the interview. If you are giving the entire structured interview, be sure to ask all the questions (except those you are specifically instructed to skip) in order to prevent errors of omission or premature diagnostic conclusions.

The 7 categories of information and the item numbers on the questionnaire are: (a) description of the symptoms, extent, and duration of insomnia (items 1–7); (b) psychological contributing factors (8–16); (c) sleep hygiene (17–27); (d) psychopathology (28–32); (e) organic sleep pathology (33–39); (f) serious medical problems (40–45); and (g) previous treatment for insomnia (46–48). If the Sleep History Questionnaire is your primary assessment tool and certain items are answered in the positive direction, these items should be pursued further by asking the indicated structured interview questions (see Table 5.3).

Table 5.2. Sleep History Questionnaire

Name _____ Date _____

1. How many nights per week do you usually have difficulty falling asleep? _____
2. On nights when you *do have* difficulty falling asleep, how many *minutes* does it usually take you to fall asleep after going to bed? _____
3. On nights when you *do not have* difficulty getting to sleep, how many *minutes* does it usually take you to fall asleep after going to bed? _____
4. Do you ever wake up in the middle of the night and have difficulty falling back to sleep?   YES   NO
   a) If yes, about how many nights does this happen each week? _____
   b) On the average, how many times do you wake up each night? _____
   c) How many minutes does it usually take you to get back to sleep each time you awaken? _____
5. How often do you wake up early in the morning, before your scheduled wake time, and are unable to return to sleep? _____
6. On nights when you have insomnia, approximately how long do you sleep each night? _____
7. How long have you had a sleep problem? _____
8. How long would you like to be able to sleep each night? _____
9. Is your sleep problem sometimes worse than other times?   YES   NO
   If yes, explain _____
   _____
10. Why do you think you have a sleep problem? _____
    _____
11. Was the onset of your problem related to any specific event?   YES   NO
    If yes, describe _____
    _____
12. Do you sleep better when you are away from home?   YES   NO
13. What do you do when you can't sleep? _____
    _____
14. When you try to sleep, is it hard for you to turn off your mind? YES   NO
15. Have you been under more stress than usual recently?   YES   NO
    If yes, explain _____
    _____
16. Are you the kind of person who tends to worry a lot?   YES   NO
17. How often is your sleep disturbed by environmental factors such as traffic, neighbors, or family members? _____
18. Is your bedroom adequately dark at night?   YES   NO
19. On weekends or your days off, do you sleep more than an hour later than your usual wake up time?   YES   NO
20. How many times per week do you take naps? _____
21. Are you on a weight loss program?   YES   NO

22. Do you engage in some kind of regular physical exercise?   YES   NO
    If yes, describe the kind, frequency, and time of day _____
23. How many cups or glasses of caffeinated beverages (e.g. coffee, tea, or cola) do
    you drink in a day?   coffee   tea   cola
24. How many days a week do you drink caffeinated beverages after 4 p.m.? _____
25. Do you take any medications that contain caffeine or stimulants (e.g., allergy
    medication or pain killers)?   YES   NO
    a) If yes, what medication and dose? _____
    b) How often do you usually take it? _____
    c) How soon before bed do you take it? _____
26. How often do you use alcohol to aid sleep? _____
27. How many cigarettes a day do you smoke? _____
28. Does difficulty sleeping ever affect your mood during the day?   YES   NO
    If yes, describe how your mood is affected _____
    _____
29. Would you describe yourself as an especially nervous person?   YES   NO
30. Estimate how many nightmares you have had in the past year _____
31. How often and what amounts of alcohol do you drink? _____
32. Have you ever been treated or hospitalized for mental, emotional, drug, or alcohol
    problems?   YES   NO
    If yes, describe _____
33. Does difficulty sleeping affect your functioning during the day?   YES   NO
    If yes, describe how it affects your functioning _____
    _____
34. Do you snore?   YES   NO
35. Do you ever wake up in the night and feel unable to breathe?   YES   NO
36. Do your legs ever jerk repeatedly or feel restless after you go to bed at
    night?   YES   NO
37. Do you ever work the night shift (11 p.m.–7 a.m.)?   YES   NO
37. How often?_____
38. Do you work a rotating or split shift?   YES   NO
    If yes, describe _____
39. Have you recently taken any prescription or over-the-counter medication for
    sleeping problems?   YES   NO
    a) If yes, what medication and amount are you taking? _____
    b) How many nights a week do you usually take this medication?_____
    c) How long have you been taking sleeping medication?_____
40. Are you currently taking any other medication?   YES   NO
    a) If yes, what medication is it? _____
    b) What illness was it prescribed for? _____
41. Do you have any other physical problems or illnesses?   YES   NO
    If yes, describe _____

42. Have you ever been hospitalized during the past 10 years?   YES   NO

    If yes, please describe _____

---

43. Have you ever had any convulsions or significant head injury?   YES   NO

    If yes, describe _____

44. How many times per night do you wake up to use the bathroom? _____

45. How many nights per week do you have indigestion or heartburn? _____

46. Have you previously received treatment for sleeping problems?   YES   NO

    If yes, describe _____

47. Have you tried any self-help remedies for your sleeping problems? YES   NO

    If yes, describe _____

48. Would you be willing to devote 30 minutes per day to a program of treatment to improve your sleep?   YES   NO

Table 5.3. Questionnaire Items to be Followed Up on the Structured Interview

Questionnaire Items	Condition to Rule Out	Interview Items
4	Depression, sleep apnea, myoclonus	5, 34–38
5	Depression	5
8	Performance anxiety, unrealistic expectations	8
11	Stress, environmental factors	15–17
12	Conditioning factors	12–13
15	Stress	15–16
16	Personality factors	8, 10, 14, 16
26	Alcohol abuse	31–32
28	Depression	5
29	Anxiety disorder	29, 32
30	Schizophrenia	30, 32
31	Alcohol abuse	31–32
32	Serious psychopathology, drug or alcohol abuse	29, 31–32
33	Sleep apnea, myoclonus	33–38
34, 35	Sleep apnea	33–37
36	Myoclonus, restless legs	38
38	Delayed sleep phase	39–42
39	Drug-induced insomnia	43
40–42	Serious physical illness	44–47
43	Neurological dysfunction	48
44	Kidney or heart disease, hypertension	4
45	Gastric reflux	50

Table 5.4. Structured Sleep History Interview

Name _____ Date _____ Interviewer _____

Please describe the problems you are having with your sleep.

1. How many nights per week do you usually have trouble sleeping?
2. How long does it usually take you to get to sleep on those nights?
3. On nights when you do *not* have trouble sleeping, how long does it usually take you to sleep?
4. Do you ever wake up in the middle of the night and have difficulty falling back to sleep? If yes,
    a) About how many nights does this happen each week?
    b) On the average, how many times do you wake up each night?
    c) How long does it usually take you to get back to sleep?
5. How often do you wake up early in the morning, before your scheduled wake time, and are unable to return to sleep? If positive,
    a) How much earlier do you awaken before your scheduled wake time?
    b) How long are you awake?
    c) Have you noticed any changes in energy level/appetite/sex drive/mood/concentration?
    If 4 or 5 are significant, rule out depression (5d–g), apnea (34–37), or myoclonus (38); if not, go to 6.
    d) How would you describe your mood lately?
    e) What are your thoughts and feelings about the future?
    f) Have you lost interest in activities that are usually pleasurable?
    g) Do your sleep problems predate feelings of depression?
    If depression is indicated, administer the Beck Depression Inventory and assess suicide potential.
6. On nights when you have insomnia, approximately how long do you sleep each night?
7. How long have you had a sleep problem?
8. How long would you like to be able to sleep each night?
    If the amount desired seems unreasonable, check for unrealistic expectations and/or performance anxiety.
    a) How much do you worry about not being able to fall or remain asleep?
9. Is your sleep problem sometimes worse than other times? If yes,
    a) How many times per month does it get bad?
    b) How long does it last?
    c) Any recent changes in your sleep problem?
10. Why do you think you have a sleep problem?
11. Was the onset of your problem related to any specific event?
    If yes, check for stress or environmental factors.
12. Do you sleep better when you are away from home?
    If yes, ask a–c to check for conditioned insomnia.
    a) How often do you fall asleep in places other than your bedroom (e.g., in front of television)?
    b) Do you have trouble regaining sleep when you move to the bedroom?
    c) Do you ever fall asleep before getting into your bedclothes?
13. What do you do when you can't sleep?
14. When you try to sleep, is it hard for you to turn off your mind? If yes,
    a) What do you usually think about?
    b) Do you ever have "racing thoughts?"
15. Have you been under more stress than usual recently?

16. Are you the kind of person who tends to worry a lot?
    If yes, rule out anxiety disorder.
17. How often is your sleep disturbed by environmental factors such as traffic, neighbors, or family members?
18. Is your bedroom adequately dark at night; is the temperature comfortable?
19. How consistent from day to day is your time to go to bed and time to get up in the morning?
    a) On weekends or your days off, do you sleep more than an hour later than your usual wake up time?
    b) Do you wake up each morning by yourself or with an alarm?
20. Do you take naps? If yes,
    a) How many days per week and how many times per day?
    b) At what time of day and is the time consistent from day to day?
    c) How long do your naps last?
    d) How long does it take you to fall asleep for a nap?
    e) Do you awake from a nap feeling refreshed or groggy?
    f) Over how long a period have you been taking naps?
21. Are you on a weight-loss program?
22. Do you engage in some kind of regular physical exercise? If yes,
    a) Describe the kind, frequency, and time of day.
23. How many cups or glasses of caffeinated beverages (e.g., coffee, tea, or cola) do you drink in a day? How much chocolate do you consume in a day?
24. How many days a week do you consume caffeine after 4 p.m.?
25. Do you take any medications that contain caffeine or stimulants (e.g., allergy medication or pain killers)? If yes,
    a) What medication and dose?
    b) How often do you usually take it?
    c) How soon before bedtime do you take it?
26. How often do you use alcohol to aid sleep?
    If yes, rule out alcohol abuse.
27. How many cigarettes a day do you smoke? After 6 p.m.?
28. Does difficulty sleeping ever affect your mood during the day? If yes,
    a) Describe how your mood is affected.
    If mood disturbance is reported, rule out depression (see 5 d–g).
29. Would you describe yourself as an especially nervous person?
    If yes, rule out anxiety disorder.
30. Estimate how many nightmares you have had in the past year.
    If more than 6 nightmares, ask a–i; if not, skip to question 31.
    a) How often do you have nightmares?
    b) How intense are they? Do they ever wake you up?
    c) Do you ever wake up screaming?
    If yes, rule out night terrors (c1–c3); if not, move to question d.
       1) Do you wake up afraid with no dream recall, or only recall a single frightening image?
       2) At these times do you notice sweating? Fast pulse?
       3) Do you ever sleepwalk?
    d) How long have you had nightmares?
    e) Any specific events or concerns that tend to elicit your nightmares?
    f) Any recurrent themes?
    If significant nightmare history, ask g–i; if not, skip to question 31.
    g) Do you ever experience vivid dreamlike scenes even though you know you are not totally asleep?
    h) Do you ever wake up and not remember who you are?
    i) Do you ever wake up and feel that someone is on the end of the bed?
    If any of g–i are positive, rule out schizophrenia.
31. Do you drink alcohol? If yes,

    a)   How often and what amounts and kinds of alcohol do you drink?
    If significant, rule out alcohol abuse.

32. Have you ever been treated or hospitalized for mental, emotional, drug, or alcohol problems?
    If positive, rule out serious psychopathology or substance abuse.

33. What effect does your sleep problem have on your daytime functioning?
    a)   How rested do you feel when you wake up?
    b)   Do you have any problems waking up?
    c)   Do you have difficulty staying awake during the day? While driving?
    d)   Has your work suffered as a result of loss of sleep?
    If substantial, rule out apnea (questions 34–37), nocturnal myoclonus (38), or delayed phase (39–42).

34. Do you snore? If yes,
    a)   Has a bedpartner ever complained of your snoring?
    b)   Is there any change in your snoring with different sleep positions?

35. What is your height/weight? (Also note client body type and neck shape.)

36. Do you ever wake up in the night and feel unable to breathe?

37. Do you ever experience shortness of breath and/or dizziness?

38. Do your legs ever bother you after you go to bed at night (e.g., cramps, jerking movements, crawling sensations)?
    If yes, rule out myoclonus or restless legs (a–g); if no, go to 39.
    a)   How long have you had this problem?
    b)   Any recent changes?
    c)   At night, do you feel like something is crawling on your legs and you have to shake it off or move your legs?
    d)   Do you ever wake up because of a cramp in your leg?
    e)   Do you ever notice that parts of your body jerk at night?
    f)   How often are the sheets pulled out from the bottom of your bed in the morning?
    g)   What do you do to relieve your leg discomfort? Does the sensation recur?

39. Do you ever work the night shift (11 p.m.–7 a.m.)? How often?

40. Do you work a rotating or split shift?

41. If you stay up late one night, do you have trouble getting to sleep the next night?

42. Do you ever get jet lag when traveling? If yes,
    a)   Do you often travel across time zones?

43. Have you recently taken any prescription or over-the-counter medication for sleeping problems, or have you recently discontinued use of these drugs?
    If yes, rule out drug-induced or rebound insomnia.
    a)   What medication and amount are you or were you taking?
    b)   How many nights a week do you usually take this medication?
    c)   How long have you been taking sleeping medication?

44. Are you currently taking any other medication? If yes,
    a)   What medication is it?
    b)   What illness was it prescribed for?

45. Do you have any other physical problems or illnesses?

46. Have you ever been hospitalized during the past 10 years?

47. Do you ever have trouble sleeping because of pain?
    If any of 44–47 are positive, rule out serious or painful medical conditions.

48. Have you ever had any convulsions or significant head injury?

49. How many times per night do you wake up to use the bathroom? If positive,
    a)   Do you have high blood pressure, heart disease, or take diuretics?

50. Do you ever have indigestion or heartburn at night?
    If significant, ask a–d to rule out gastric reflux; if not, skip to 51.
    a)   Describe your history with this problem.
    b)   Do certain foods keep you awake?
    c)   Do you take anything for the problem; does it relieve the symptoms?
    d)   Do you ever wake up with nausea or with vomit in your mouth?

51. Have you previously received treatment for sleeping problems?
52. Have you tried any self-help remedies for your sleeping problems?
53. Would you be willing to devote 30 minutes per day to a program of treatment to improve your sleep?

In addition to interviewing the poor sleeper, many researchers find it helpful to question the client's bedpartner to elicit history that may be helpful in making a diagnosis of organic sleep pathology. In particular, the bedpartner should be asked questions about snoring, abnormal motor activity during sleep, unusual daytime sleepiness, and nap taking.

PSYCHOLOGICAL INVENTORIES

The experience of disrupted sleep is often associated with mood changes, anxiety, tense and obsessive personality style, and psychopathology, especially depression. To aid in the total assessment of the person complaining of insomnia, sleep researchers often turn to various psychological inventories. The most frequently used measure of this type is the MMPI for the description of personality and diagnosis of psychopathology. If depression is suspected, then the Beck Depression Inventory (Beck, 1967) can be useful. An important point to remember is that not only can depression be the primary diagnosis, with sleep difficulties among the symptoms of the depression, but that insomnia may develop first and over time cause the person to come to feel hopeless, helpless, and demoralized. Also, be aware that many depression inventories include sleep disturbance items that may spuriously raise the depression scores of individuals who suffer from insomnia. It is important to ascertain whether the course of the sleep problems paralleled the course of the mood disturbance or if the sleep problems pre-dated the depression. In the latter case, the sleep problems tend to persist even when the mood disturbance fluctuates from week to week.

Other kinds of psychological inventories that can be useful in the assessment of sleep disturbance are those that focus on stress (Hassles and Uplifts scales, Kanner, Coyne, Schaefer, & Lazarus, 1981; Psychosomatic Symptom Checklist, Cox, Freundlich, & Meyer, 1975), anxiety (State-Trait Anxiety Inventory, Spielberger, Gorsuch, & Lushene, 1970), mood (Profile of Mood States, Pillard, Atkinson, & Fisher, 1967), medical complaints and attributions (Multidimensional Health Locus of Control Scale, K. A. Wallston, B. S. Wallston, & DeVellis, 1978), and life satisfaction (Philadelphia Geriatric Center Morale Scale, Lawton, 1972). In addition to using psychological inventories before treatment begins, some of these inventories may be repeated following the therapy or at follow-up to measure the effectiveness of the intervention.

SLEEP DIARY

The purpose of the daily sleep diary is to monitor continuously the subjective complaint of insomnia. The diary provides an inexpensive, nonintrusive, and efficient method of measuring the experiential component of insomnia, which is the usual impetus for the insomniac to seek treatment. The exact origin of the particular sleep diary format is unknown. Researchers and clinicians originally used retrospective questionnaires for subjects to describe the extent of their sleep problems. However, that type of assessment is notoriously subject to all kinds of biases. Therefore, responses on the Sleep History Questionnaire regarding the amount of sleep lost at night should be taken only as very general estimates, not as baseline levels of the target behaviors. In the early 1970s insomnia researchers gradually switched to sleep diaries to provide continuous daily monitoring of the target behaviors associated with insomnia. Use of daily sleep diaries is the current standard for work in this area and provides rich detail of the client's sleep patterns. The content for many of the questions on the sleep diary derives to a large extent from Monroe's research (1967). Content and format have been remarkably consistent across studies, enabling researchers to build a data base and to compare results across investigations.

In our own research we have added the requirement that participants must mail their sleep diaries to us each day. Each week of treatment they are given 7 prestamped and addressed diaries. In this way we can ensure monitoring on a daily basis and greatly reduce the possibility of retrospective estimates. Clients complete the diary upon awakening and mail it every day during baseline, treatment, and follow-up, giving us a screening, intervention, and maintenance measure of the target behavior. We have used this diary successfully with hundreds of participants and have had no problems with their understanding of it or with client compliance in returning the diaries every morning.

On the sleep diary (see Table 5.5) clients are asked to record, soon after awakening, their estimate in minutes of their sleep onset latency (SOL) the previous night. They also indicate the number and lengths of awakenings during the night in order to allow calculation of wake time after sleep onset (WASO) and the total amount of sleep for the night. Some rigid and obsessive clients become concerned about providing exact calculations of time. To prevent exacerbation of performance anxiety they must not become clock watchers but just try to give their best estimate. Absolute accuracy is not essential. Participants are also asked to rate, on a 5-point scale, 6 items regarding the quality of their sleep and of their daytime functioning. Sleep researchers sometimes

Table 5.5. Daily Sleep Diary

Name _____ Date _____
1. How many minutes did it take you to fall asleep last night?_____
2. How many times did you awaken during the night?_____
3. Please record how long you were awake (in minutes) for each occurrence listed
   above in question number 2.

   _____   _____   _____

   _____   _____   _____

   _____   _____   _____

4. What is the total number of hours and minutes you slept last night? _____
5. How difficult was it for you to fall asleep last night?

   1   2   3   4   5
   Not very   Extremely
   difficult   difficult
6. How rested do you feel this morning?

   1   2   3   4   5
   Very rested   Poorly rested
7. Rate the quality of last night's sleep.

   1   2   3   4   5
   Excellent   Very poor
8. What was your level of physical tension when you went to bed last night?

   1   2   3   4   5
   Extremely   Extremely tense
   relaxed
9. Rate your level of mental activity when you went to bed last night.

   1   2   3   4   5
   Very quiet   Very active
10. How well do you think you were functioning yesterday?

   1   2   3   4   5
   Very well   Very poorly

Please Fold, Secure and Mail Daily

---

also include a question about the amount and kind of sleep-inducing medication used the previous night. If you have required the client to forego drugs during behavior therapy or if the client has never used drugs for sleep you may wish to follow our practice of omitting this item.

Normative studies have established clearcut differences in subjectively reported SOL between insomniacs and good sleepers. In 8 studies of good sleepers ($n = 134$), subjective SOL ranged from 9 to 14 minutes (mean = 12.6) when the person slept at home and from 15 to 38 minutes (mean = 24.6) when sleep was in a laboratory. Seven sleep laboratory studies of insomniacs ($n = 217$) also collected sleep diary data; SOLs ranged from 37 to 81 minutes (mean = 56.7) (Lacks, in press). In a 1978 review of 7 treatment studies of clinical cases of insomnia the mean SOL was 82 minutes (Bootzin & Nicassio). The mean baseline sleep complaint for 216 participants in 7 outcome studies conducted in our research program was 72 minutes SOL and 88 minutes WASO (Lacks & Powlishta, 1986). Little is known about subjective estimates of other aspects of sleep for good sleepers but 2 studies have reported the following figures for insomnia sufferers: 67 minutes for WASO (Coates et al., 1982; Lichstein, Nickel, Hoelscher, & Kelley, 1982) and 330 total minutes of sleep (Carskadon et al., 1976; Frankel, Coursey, Buchbinder, & Snyder, 1976).

In addition to these mean values of self-report of sleep, behavior therapists should be aware of the high night-to-night variability of the sleep of insomnia sufferers. Total sleep diary variance for poor sleepers has been shown to exceed by a considerable amount the variance for good sleepers. Many sleep researchers think that it is this variability rather than the short sleep itself that is the major source of the insomniac's complaint of daytime dysphoria. Because of this variability, it is important to ensure sufficient sampling over time of the insomniac's sleep behavior. Probably 2 weeks is the ideal amount of time for baseline monitoring. Many individuals who have suffered from chronic insomnia for years can have occasional good weeks that coincide with baseline measurement. It is our own practice to consider the first week to be one of adaptation to the measure and to consider the second week as our pretreatment or baseline level of the target behavior. Do not start monitoring sleep with daily diaries until the client has been drug free at least 2 or preferably 3 weeks.

Even though there are many potential sources of bias with such a self-report, research on the subjective estimate as recorded on a specific-item daily sleep diary has generally been very favorable. This finding is in marked contrast to results with more global and/or retrospective sleep questionnaires. Test-retest reliability is high. In one study the average test-retest reliability for SOL was .86. Another found .93 for poor sleepers and .58 for good sleepers. Agreement across 3 nights was found to be .98 for SOL, .88 for number of arousals, and .84 for WASO (Bootzin & Engle-Friedman, 1981).

Measures of validity are equally encouraging. Subjective estimates of SOL from insomniacs have been found to correlate very highly with spouse or roommate observer estimates (*rs* ranging from .84 to .99). Another researcher found high correspondence between self-report of SOL, observor estimate, and a clock that insomniacs activated with a switch in bed (Franklin, 1981). This parallel relationship between sleep diary and the clock only occurred during the second week of the experiment after a significant reduction occurred in subjective SOL between the first and second weeks. Insomniacs may need a week of practice to develop consistency in estimating SOL. Using student poor sleepers, other researchers found the correlation between subjective estimate and EEG to increase from .37 on the second night in the laboratory to .75 by the fourth night (Freedman & Papsdorf, 1976). From these studies, it would appear that insomniacs should be given 1 week to develop estimation accuracy before baseline figures are collected in the second week. Converging evidence points to insomniacs as being better estimators of the phenomenology of sleep than are good sleepers, perhaps because insomniacs have many years of experience observing the target behavior (Bootzin & Engle-Friedman, 1981).

A number of researchers have verified with all-night polysomnography (EEG) insomniacs' subjective reports of improvement following therapy. SOLs have also been found to correlate highly with EEG estimates (rs ranging from .62 to .99) with the higher values occurring when more conservative criteria for sleep onset are used. Correlations between EEG and other diary items are generally lower: number of arousals (rs ranging from .27 to .63), WASO (rs = .83 to .88), and total sleep time (rs=.42 and .64) (Lacks, in press).

Much of the criticism of subjective SOL is that these estimates are an overestimate of awake time compared with EEG measures and to ratings by observers. Studies have shown a consistent and constant 10 to 25 minutes subjective overestimation of time to fall asleep using the EEG as the objective criterion. However, as already discussed in chapter 2, it may be that for insomniacs the experience of sleep onset actually occurs at a later time during the EEG-assessed transition from waking to sleeping. It may be that the self-report estimate is closer to the experienced sleep onset than are the traditional EEG markers of sleep onset.

OBJECTIVE SLEEP MEASURES

For most practitioners, the subjective sleep diary will provide sufficient information to monitor treatment progress. Reseachers in this area, however, may want to consider some more objective measure of sleep. In the past, the only alternative has been assessment by polysomnography within a sleep laboratory. This method, although empirical, is expensive, not always available, and may not give an accurate picture of the way a person sleeps at home. Recently, however, researchers who have wanted to monitor the outcome of treatment for insomnia in the natural environment have developed an inexpensive, convenient, switch-activated clock. While awake, subjects hold down a switch connected to a clock that operates continuously as long as the switch is pressed. When subjects fall asleep the relaxation of the thumb pressure releases the switch and leaves the clock displaying the SOL. Morin et al. (1986) found good correspondence between self-report and a similar electromechanical timer for 27 elderly persons with sleep maintenance problems (SOL $rs = .87$ and $.95$, WASO $rs = .65$ and $.97$ at baseline and posttreatment, respectively).

Kelley and Lichstein (1980) have developed a more expensive method that consists of a series of solid-state timers, a tone generator that operates every 10 minutes throughout the night, and a tape recorder that is activated briefly with each tone to capture any response if the subject is awake. Researchers then have a record of sleep status at 10-minute intervals and can extrapolate amounts of time awake. Comparisons with EEG showed validity coefficients of $.83$ for stage 1 sleep and $.94$ for stage 2 sleep and correlations with self-reports of $.97$.

SPECIALIZED MEASURES TO USE WITH INSOMNIA

There are a number of specialized measures of behaviors and attitudes associated with sleep disturbance. Three that may be particularly helpful in assessing sleep problems and in measuring treatment effectiveness deal with (a) sleep hygiene, (b) cognitive and somatic arousal, and (c) self-efficacy.

The Sleep Hygiene Awareness and Practice Scale (SHAPS) was developed for our research to assess the extent of the poor sleeper's awareness of sleep hygiene principles and how frequently these principles are applied (Lacks & Rotert, 1986). The SHAPS is presented in Table 5.6; scoring instructions can be found in the Appendix. The Hygiene Knowledge section contains items on general sleep hygiene awareness, that is, whether specific activities are seen as beneficial to sleep, disruptive to sleep, or as having no effect. All the listed activities are known to have an effect on sleep. In the Caffeine Knowledge section, common foods, beverages, and nonprescription drugs are listed and the client is asked to indicate whether the substance contains caffeine. The Hygiene Practice section contains questions asking how many nights per week the client typically engages in the same items of behavior from the knowledge section, plus items asking about disturbance of sleep from worry, noise, light, temperature, and bedpartner. Answers to individual questions can also aid the therapist in planning what sleep hygiene material needs to be covered during treatment.

Many insomnia sufferers complain of racing thoughts or cognitive arousal at bedtime; fewer report that they experience somatic tension or

Table 5.6. Sleep Hygiene Awareness and Practice Scale

Name _____ Date _____

Sleep Hygiene Knowledge
This is a survey of the effect of selected daytime behaviors upon sleep. We are interested in knowing your opinion about whether any of these daytime behaviors influence the quality and/or quantity of sleep. For the following list of behaviors, please indicate your opinion as to the extent of the general effect, if any, that each behavior may have on nightly sleep. Please use the following scale and answer each item by writing the appropriate number in the space provided. Note that numbers 1, 2, and 3 indicate degrees of *benefit* to sleep, number 4 indicates *no effect* on sleep, and numbers 5, 6, and 7 indicate degrees of *disruption* of sleep.

	Beneficial to sleep		No effect		Disruptive to sleep	
1	2	3	4	5	6	7
very	moderately	mildly		mildly	moderately	very

What effect do each of these behaviors have upon sleep?
1. Daytime napping _____
2. Going to bed hungry _____
3. Going to bed thirsty _____
4. Smoking more than one pack of cigarettes a day _____
5. Using sleep medication regularly (prescription or over-the-counter) _____
6. Exercising strenuously within 2 hours of bedtime _____
7. Sleeping approximately the same length of time each night _____
8. Setting aside time to relax before bedtime _____
9. Consuming food, beverages, or medications containing caffeine _____
10. Exercising in the afternoon or early evening _____
11. Waking up at the same time each day _____
12. Going to bed at the same time each day _____
13. Drinking 3 ounces of alcohol in the evening (e.g., 3 mixed drinks, 3 beers, 3 glasses of wine) _____

Caffeine Knowledge
For each item on the following list, indicate whether you believe it contains caffeine or another stimulant by placing a Y (yes) or an N (no) in the space provided. If you are not sure, make your best guess. If you have never heard of an item please place an X in the space.

___ 7-Up soft drink	___ lemonade	___ Mountain Dew
___ regular tea	___ root beer	___ cola soft drinks
___ Dristan cold remedy	___ chocolate cake	___ Dexatrim diet pills
___ aspirin	___ regular coffee	___ Tylenol
___ Dr. Pepper soft drink	___ Excedrin	___ Aqua Ban diuretic
___ Midol menstrual relief	___ Sudafed decongestant	___ Sprite soft drink

Sleep Hygiene Practice
For each of the following behaviors state the number of days per week (0–7) that you engage in that activity or have that experience. Base your answers on what you would consider an average week for yourself.

Indicate the number of days or nights in an average week you:
1. Take a nap_____
2. Go to bed hungry_____
3. Go to bed thirsty_____
4. Smoke more than one pack of cigarettes_____
5. Use sleeping medications (prescription or over-the-counter)_____
6. Drink beverages containing caffeine (e.g., coffee, tea, colas) within 4 hours of bedtime_____
7. Drink more than 3 ounces of alcohol (e.g., 3 mixed drinks, 3 beers, or 3 glasses of wine) within 2 hours of bedtime_____
8. Take medications/drugs with caffeine within 4 hours of bedtime_____
9. Worry as you prepare for bed about your ability to sleep_____
10. Worry during the day about your ability to sleep at night_____
11. Use alcohol to facilitate sleep_____
12. Exercise strenuously within 2 hours of bedtime_____
13. Have your sleep disturbed by light_____
14. Have your sleep disturbed by noise_____
15. Have your sleep disturbed by your bedpartner_____ (put NA if no partner)
16. Sleep approximately the same length of time each night_____
17. Set aside time to relax before bedtime_____
18. Exercise in the afternoon or early evening_____
19. Have a comfortable nighttime temperature in your bed/bedroom_____

---

arousal. However, optimal treatment planning will be facilitated by some knowledge of whether the client is having a significant problem with either cognitive or somatic arousal or a combination of both. Nicassio and his colleagues at Vanderbilt University have recently developed the Pre-Sleep Arousal Scale (PSAS) (Nicassio et al., 1985) to assess this phenomenology in the presleep state. The PSAS is made up of 8 somatic and 8 cognitive items combined to make a single 16-item scale (see Table 5.7). The ratings on the 5-point scale are added for the somatic items (numbers, 1, 2, 5, 7, 10, 12, 13, 15), the cognitive items (numbers 3, 4, 6, 8, 9, 11, 14, 16), and for a combined score. Normative data can be found in the 1985 paper.

Following behavior therapy for insomnia, one of the most dramatic changes is an increase in clients' perceptions of self-efficacy, or their ability to exercise influence over their own sleep-related motivation and behavior. Repeatedly, on follow-up questionnaires, our research subjects verbalized that although they did not feel they had been "cured" of

Table 5.7. Pre-Sleep Arousal Scale

Name _____ Date _____

During the pre-sleep period last night (in bed with the lights out before falling asleep for the first time), did you have any of the following experiences? Please indicate (by circling the appropriate number) the degree to which you experienced each of those listed below. Do not include what you experienced during the middle of the night if you awakened after falling asleep.

		Not at all	A little	Moder- ately	A lot	Extremely
1.	Heart racing, pounding, or beating irregularly	1	2	3	4	5
2.	A jittery, nervous feeling in your body	1	2	3	4	5
3.	Worry about falling asleep	1	2	3	4	5
4.	Review or ponder events of the day	1	2	3	4	5
5.	Shortness of breath or labored breathing	1	2	3	4	5
6.	Depressing or anxious thoughts	1	2	3	4	5
7.	A tight, tense feeling in your muscles	1	2	3	4	5
8.	Worry about problems other than sleep	1	2	3	4	5
9.	Being mentally alert, active	1	2	3	4	5
10.	Cold feeling in your hands, feet, or your body in general	1	2	3	4	5
11.	Can't shut off your thoughts	1	2	3	4	5
12.	Have stomach upset (knot or nervous feeling in stomach, heartburn, nausea, gas, etc.)	1	2	3	4	5
13.	Perspiration in palms of your hands or other parts of your body	1	2	3	4	5
14.	Thoughts keep running through your head	1	2	3	4	5
15.	Dry feeling in mouth or throat	1	2	3	4	5
16.	Distracted by sounds, noise in the environment (e.g., ticking clock, house noises, traffic)	1	2	3	4	5

Note: From "The phenomenology of the pre-sleep state: The development of the Pre-Sleep Arousal Scale" by P. M. Nicassio, D. R. Mendlowitz, J. J. Fussell, and L. Petras, 1985, Behaviour Research and Therapy, 23, 266. Copyright 1985 by Perry Nicassio. Reprinted by permission.

insomnia, they no longer felt they were helpless to do anything about it. Their sleep problems were improved but they still expected to have occasional future bouts of sleep disturbance. However, they now felt confident they would not panic when such bouts occurred; they had techniques to implement; and they would be able to keep occasional sleep problems from becoming chronic and debilitating.

Because these informal reports were so frequent and seemed to represent large changes, we developed a Self-Efficacy Scale (Table 5.8) to document them using ideas from Bootzin (Bootzin et al., 1983). This scale (with possible scores ranging from 9 to 45) can be given at baseline and again at the end of treatment or at follow-up after clients have had a longer time to practice their new behaviors. Although we have not published normative data, the results from M. A. Cook and Lacks (1984) are representative of what we have found in several studies. For 28 sleep onset insomniacs who received stimulus control therapy, average perceived self-efficacy went from 23.5 to 33.

MEDICAL AND SLEEP LABORATORY EVALUATION

A thorough assessment of any complaint of sleep disturbance should include a complete physical history and medical examination by the client's physician. Such a precaution is necessary because some complaints of sleep problems can be due to a medical condition or to organic sleep pathology. The examining physician should be asked to determine the extent to which physical condition and current medications may be contributing to the client's sleep disturbance. Guidelines for deciding whether to make a referral to a specialized sleep disorders center were included in chapter 3. If you suspect that the client has sleep apnea, nocturnal myoclonus, restless legs, or narcolepsy, only evaluation through polysomnography can confirm or rule out your suspicions. If you do refer the client to a sleep disorders center, a physical examination will be included as a standard part of that evaluation.

Table 5.8. Self-Efficacy Scale

_____

Name _____Date _____

For the following 9 items, please rate (by circling a number from 1 to 5) your ability to carry out each behavior. If you feel able to accomplish a behavior some of the time but not always, you should indicate a lower level of confidence.

Indicate how confident you are that you can:

1. Lie in bed, feeling physically relaxed.
         1   2   3   4   5
    Not confident   Very confident
      at all

2. Lie in bed, feeling mentally relaxed.
         1   2   3   4   5
    Not confident   Very confident
      at all

3. Lie in bed with your thoughts "turned off."
         1   2   3   4   5
    Not confident   Very confident
      at all

4. Fall asleep at night in under 30 minutes.
         1   2   3   4   5
    Not confident   Very confident
      at all

5. Wake up at night fewer than 3 times.
         1   2   3   4   5
    Not confident   Very confident
      at all

6. Go back to sleep within 15 minutes of waking in the night.
         1   2   3   4   5
    Not confident   Very confident
      at all

7. Feel refreshed upon waking in the morning.
         1   2   3   4   5
    Not confident   Very confident
      at all

8. Wake after a poor night's sleep without feeling upset about it.
         1   2   3   4   5
    Not confident   Very confident
      at all

9. Not allow a poor night's sleep to interfere with daily activities.
         1   2   3   4   5
    Not confident   Very confident
      at all

Chapter 6
Overview of Stimulus Control Treatment for Insomnia

The behavioral strategies for the alleviation of persistent insomnia that will be described in this chapter are organized within a highly structured format of lessons, group discussion, and questions and answers. It is our experience that the goals of this particular kind of therapy can best be accomplished in a group format; however, the procedures can be modified for treatment of individuals. Ordinarily, if the therapist can maintain control of the process, the therapy can be completed in four or five sessions of about an hour each with 90 minutes for the first session. Control of the treatment process means working actively within a closely defined structure to guide and influence the pace and direction of the therapy. This treatment is not open ended or nondirective. The approximately 400 insomnia sufferers treated by our research team tended to be well educated, psychologically minded, and familiar with an educational approach and the concept of record keeping. If many of the participants are older adults or of average intelligence, six sessions may be preferable to allow a slower pace and more repetition of important points. The treatment to be described is a multifaceted approach including the following therapeutic elements:

- The therapist
- Group process
- Sleep education
- Self-monitoring
- Self-control and reduction of performance anxiety
- Sleep hygiene

- Specific techniques
- Additional optional techniques

Each of these elements will now be discussed before the actual therapy sessions are described in the next 2 chapters.

THE THERAPIST AS A TREATMENT COMPONENT

Although it may seem self-evident, the therapist plays a key and specific role in this behavioral treatment of insomnia. As was discussed in the beginning of the book, group members expect the therapist to be quite knowledgeable about sleep and insomnia. Having this knowledge about sleep, its disorders, and their alleviation will be essential to help the therapist "hook" the client into treatment. The goal is to move the client from a passive, pill-taking mode to a problem-solving, self-reliant mode. You can imagine that it would be difficult to convince someone to give up sleeping pills if you did not know why hypnotics are undesirable and ineffective. Clients need to feel that they have come to the right place to get relief from their sleep disturbance. Programs such as this one have been very succesful in alleviating the sleep problems of many people. To accomplish this goal, the therapist will have to appear self-confident, knowledgeable, experienced, organized, optimistic, and as though he or she has a plan. The therapist should be able to convey clearly the rationale for the therapy, the course it will take, and the degree and schedule of expected improvement. The therapist should believe and communicate full expectations for helping clients to eliminate or to greatly improve their insomnia. The goal is for clients to see this treatment as logical and to have confidence that it will be successful for them.

On top of being expert, the therapist needs to be human in order to be successful with this kind of behavior therapy. Appearing normal and reasonable, using a touch of humor to lighten the atmosphere, avoiding jargon whenever possible, and being patient with clients' quirks and frailties will go a long way toward a successful outcome. With only 4 sessions, rapport needs to develop immediately, not after 1 or 2 sessions. A technique that can be useful in promotion of bonding with clients is the judicious use of self-disclosure. By comfortably and naturally revealing appropriate personal material, the therapist not only appears more human but also models the type of openness that clients are being encouraged to engage in within the group. The therapist is also modeling a problem-solving, coping stance. Many of my own clients have remarked that it was important to them to find out that I too had experienced problems in life and that I had been able to solve them. In the treatment of insomnia, one of the most effective pieces of self-disclosure can be the therapist's personal history of poor sleep and how it was overcome. This is not to say that therapists should fabricate a history of poor sleep, but most of us have had some brief episodes in which our sleep was disrupted, at least giving us credibility for knowing firsthand about the nighttime frustration and the next-day consequences.

Because this treatment package needs to be so structured to be completed in 4 weeks, the therapist has to keep things very much on track. Of course group discussion is allowed, and in fact is an integral part of the process; but it must be controlled, guided, and always made to enhance, not detract from or become tangential to, the proceedings. The therapist has to play the directive role of group leader and facilitator, or as one of our therapists described it, "symphony conductor." In addition, the therapist will be the one who gives feedback to clients, compliments their efforts, highlights their successes, and encourages continued problem solving.

GROUP PROCESS

Some researchers have found no differences in outcome between behavior therapy provided in small groups and that provided to individuals (e.g., Teri & Lewinsohn, 1986, for treatment of depression). Consequently, in the interests of cost efficiency, they recommend the group delivery. In our own experience, however, results with the group format appear to be far superior to those achieved by treating one person at a time. We originally chose the group format because we did not have adequate research funds to provide enough therapists for individual treatment. We thought that one-on-one procedures would naturally be the most effective way to operate but fiscally we were unable to do so. Throughout the time we were conducting research, however, there were occasional clients who could not be accommodated into a group for reasons such as time schedules or their not wanting to be placed on a waiting list. These clients were treated privately and individually using the same procedures of the therapy protocol with the exception of the group process. As far as we could tell, the individually treated clients did not differ in any way from the clients who were treated in groups. Yet the latter participants appeared to profit more from treatment than the former.

In discussions of the reasons for these paradoxical findings we concluded that the group experience provided several advantages, most importantly the element of accountability. When individually seen clients did not self-monitor properly or did not follow treatment instructions, the therapist would discuss the importance of adherence to the treatment protocol and would try to increase motivation to comply during the upcoming week. However, in the group setting, the same nonadhering client met with a more forceful reaction from other group members. Group members were less willing to tolerate nonadherence from each other. The prevailing attitude seemed to be, "If I can adhere, you sure can also. If I follow the treatment program and I see improvement, then if you do so, you will also see similar gains." The therapist can also work to facilitate this kind of response from the group members. If a client is going to be seen on an individual basis, the therapist should try to find a way to implement a similar lack of tolerance for noncompliance with the treatment procedures.

After our participants completed their treatment, we sought feedback about their progress and their reactions to the therapy experience. One of the most frequently voiced comments was that the clients found the group meetings valuable. Although insomnia is a prevalent health problem, it is surprising that many poor sleepers do not know how widespread sleep problems are in our society. It was important for our clients to meet other reasonable, seemingly normal people who had suffered for many years from poor sleep and its attendant consequences. They found it very relieving to know that they were not alone and that they were not "crazy." Furthermore, it was a relief to realize that it was acceptable to seek help for such a problem, not a sign of personal weakness. Participants also stated that they benefited greatly from the catharsis of talking about their sleep problems in a supportive atmosphere. We found this group reaction so powerful that these groups tended, with little help from the therapist, to develop a quick sense of camaraderie, cohesion, and friendship.

Because the group process has proved to be so important to this particular treatment and/or to this specific target group, the therapist needs to promote it actively as part of the intervention. The therapist should try to counteract any tendency to want to leap in with advice or to give an opinion before the group has been encouraged to do so. As an example, if a client reported difficulty carrying out one of the therapy instructions, the therapist might be tempted to suggest alternative behaviors. One result of this quickness to be therapeutic might be that other group members will then be reluctant to share their ideas because the expert has already given the "correct" answer. Also, the client having difficulty may dismiss the suggestion of the therapist as unrealistic or too difficult to implement, a resistance tactic that is harder to sustain if the suggestion has come from another client. The philosophy of the therapist should be that when it comes to problem solving, six heads are better than one. It is going to be a collaborative effort; therefore each person should plan to be actively involved. All members, not only the most verbal or dominant ones, should be expected to and shaped to participate. To make participation a safe activity, the therapist will also have to ensure that each client shows respect for the others' points of view.

From our experience, the ideal group size is 5 to 7 members. Fewer people makes it more difficult to foster support among the participants. A larger number is hard for the therapist to manage and may leave group members feeling shortchanged of individual attention. We have also found it advantageous to have relatively homogeneous groups at least with respect to background and type of sleep problem. However, we have successfully mixed males and females and younger and older adults. The inexperienced group therapist should read some additional material on the special issues of the group approach (e.g., Merritt & Walley, 1977).

BASIC SLEEP EDUCATION

Even though a good deal of information about sleep has been available through the popular media in recent years, many poor sleepers are lacking in basic knowledge about the processes and functions of sleep. They also often hold misconceptions about sleep. Therefore, one of the early tasks of the therapist will be to provide a brief and basic sleep education. Knowledge alone can be effective in alleviating performance anxiety. Furthermore, obtaining this knowledge allows the insomniac to begin to view sleep disturbance as a problem that one can cope with. The idea is that sleep is a basic and natural physiological process just like any other. As such, its natural patterns can be interfered with through a number of avenues, but there also exist a number of options for restoring its normal functioning.

Many poor sleepers think that they are victims, at the mercy of some unknown, mysterious phenomenon over which there is no possibility of gaining any control. For years they have developed a pattern of increasing tension and preoccupation with their lack of control over what seems to be such a simple and automatic process for so many others. They also are preoccupied with the negative daytime consequences of lack of sleep. Just as focusing on pain increases its subjective intensity, dwelling on feelings of fatigue can result in a similar inflation of its negative aspects. One primary goal of basic sleep education is to alter the poor sleeper's appraisal of the problem. Providing such information and support alone can have therapeutic effects by allowing the client to put the problem in a coping context (Bootzin et al., 1983). The information contained in the first few chapters of this book as well as in the suggested readings should be helpful in preparing the therapist. In general, this information should be spread somewhat naturally throughout the sessions rather than be delivered as one long boring lecture and should serve as a basis for the therapist to answer clients' questions about sleep and insomnia.

In addition to information contained elsewhere in this book such as the disruptive effect of sleep medications, the importance of sleep hygiene, and the need for sleep scheduling, we typically try to convey information about the following 6 areas:

1. Large-scale surveys have found that 15% to 36% of Americans suffer from insomnia as a current problem, with many more having had this experience at some time in their lives. At least 30 million Americans have difficulty falling or staying asleep and as a result feel tired the following day. The insomnia sufferer is not alone!

2. The belief that everyone must have a full 8 hours of sleep every night is a myth. There are large individual differences in the amount of sleep needed on a regular basis to feel refreshed. In general, if nothing is done to interfere, the body will obtain the amount of sleep that it needs to function optimally. The range of "normal" sleep varies between 3 and 10 hours per night. Some people who believe they have insomnia do not. Instead, they have made themselves tense and anguished (a state that itself can cause fatigue) trying to obtain an amount of sleep that they do not need and that their body resists. As an example, one of the first clients we treated was a woman who was averaging 3 hours per night to fall asleep. She looked very fatigued and was feeling frustrated and despondent. As treatment unfolded, it became apparent that she was not an insomniac but was instead a natural short sleeper. She really needed only 3 hours of sleep a night but was wearing herself out trying to force herself to sleep when her body did not need it. She opted instead to spend several hours at night relaxing while listening to music, eventually drifting off for a period of about 3 hours of sound sleep. Though she was spending about the same amount of time in bed both awake and asleep, her appraisal of the situation was entirely different; she was relaxed instead of anxious, and she felt restored in the morning. For this type of person, we usually emphasize the advantages of not needing so much sleep. Many of us yearn for more hours in the day to get things done and engage in pleasurable activities. Often the quiet, undisturbed hours

of late night or early morning are the ideal times to do these things.

3. The normal sleep cycle consists of periods of both light and deep sleep. Within this cycle, it is common for people to reach a point of wakefulness on the average of 4 to 5 times a night. Therefore, waking up in the middle of the night is normal. Everyone does it and most people just return to sleep fairly quickly after this brief (up to 10 minutes) surfacing. Many poor sleepers cause themselves needless anxiety by believing that their problem is waking up in the night, an experience that they think good sleepers do not have. The problem with the sleep maintenance insomniac is not usually the awakening in the night but is the difficulty in falling back asleep. This person has developed behavior that interferes with returning to sleep. Often the starting point for these sleep-incompatible behaviors was anxiety about middle-of-the-night awakenings.

4. Poor sleepers are also often unaware of the relationship of age to sleep. As a person gets older, there appears to be a natural developmental pattern of needing less sleep and awakening more often. For many insomniacs poor sleep does not develop until middle age and may be related to their attempts to achieve the same amount and quality of sleep as in their younger years. Just as a 14-year-old does not need as much sleep as a 6-year-old, so a 60-year-old may not need as much as someone who is 25.

5. Another important issue concerns the popular misconceptions about the effects of sleep deprivation. There are a number of public examples of individuals going for many days without any sleep and still being able to function normally during the daytime though maybe not as comfortably. Although most of us will feel tired and grouchy after a loss of several hours of sleep, that is about the extent of the consequences. In other words, the human body has a remarkable tolerance for loss of sleep, at least on a temporary basis. What this means to the poor sleeper is that an inadequate night's sleep is not a catastrophe or the end of the world. We usually feel tired and irritable when we have a cold but most of us manage to muddle through the next few days without becoming preoccupied about our cold or worrying about the next time we might get a cold. Clients need to be tolerant of the occasional sleeplessness that everyone experiences. A night of poor sleep is nothing to be particularly concerned about. In fact, overconcern about missed sleep is the surest route to increasingly disturbed sleep.

6. The final message that we try to convey to our clients is that there can be a behavioral basis for the development of chronic sleep troubles. There are numerous "legitimate" causes of an occasional brief bout of poor sleep. The most frequent of these is probably some kind of stress. However, when insomnia becomes persistent,

usually some process is operating other than that which caused the original sleeplessness. The chronic insomniac has developed some pattern of sleep-incompatible habits. Therefore, the treatments that we use to counteract poor sleep may not appear to the client to relate to the original cause of the sleep problem. We work instead on treating those habits that maintain the poor sleep. Our goal is not to prevent occasional sleeplessness, but rather to prevent the development of chronic sleep problems.

SLEEP MONITORING

Clients must understand that the diaries, homework logs, and other forms they fill out are not idle recordkeeping or solely a means for the therapist to track the participant's progress. These records are a part of the therapeutic process. In other words, keeping a record of sleep and related behaviors is one of the key ingredients in behavioral therapy for insomnia. Numerous studies have documented the benefits of self-monitoring upon behavior change and we believe that it plays an important role in the alleviation of poor sleep. Therefore, the therapist needs to stress the importance of accurate daily monitoring and should not tolerate any lapses or sloppiness in recordkeeping. Clients can be told that it is a tedious, though not time-consuming, task that will affect their progress in treatment. We require that clients send in their sleep diaries daily each morning so that they are not tempted to make retrospective reports (see chapter 5). The therapist or designated assistant should monitor the receipt of these diaries so that they can be scanned easily before each group session. The therapist should observe progress or lack of it, read the comments that are often written onto the diaries, and watch for errors in the monitoring procedures. The homework logs should be brought to each session and the therapist should take a few minutes to review them before the meeting starts. The fact that the therapist will be observing their self-monitoring should be conveyed to clients as an additional incentive to fill out the forms in a timely and accurate fashion.

There are at least 3 aspects of the self-monitoring that contribute to the treatment process. First, by recording sleep and other behaviors, clients become aware in a more objective way of what their sleep patterns are really like. Clients who swear and truly believe that they typically get only an hour or two of sleep a night will often find that their actual amount is somewhat higher. Clients can also see their progress as the therapy unfolds. Second, having to keep a homework log of behaviors that you are supposed to engage in, such as getting out of bed after a 10-minute period of sleeplessness, makes it more likely that you will actually follow through. In this case, the monitoring promotes adherence to the therapy. Additionally, having such records helps the client to adopt the role of "personal scientist" (e.g., Mahoney, 1977). The material can serve as data for troubleshooting when problems with implementing the therapy are encountered.

DEVELOPING A SENSE OF SELF-CONTROL

One of the most frustrating aspects of persistent insomnia is the feeling of not having control over a very important aspect of one's life. Much of the performance anxiety observed in chronic insomniacs is probably a byproduct of attempts to increase control over sleep. By the time an individual seeks out behavior therapy of poor sleep, he or she may have a lengthy history of feelings of impotence. The most frequently expressed outcome by clients in our program has been the transformation from feeling one is a helpless victim to a sense of being in charge and control again. In other words, our participants leave the program with greatly increased feelings of self-efficacy and reduced performance anxiety. This finding is not surprising given that perceived self-efficacy has been shown to play an important role in other health-related behaviors like smoking cessation relapse, pain management, and weight control (O'Leary, 1985).

Interestingly, this increased sense of personal capability occurs regardless of whether sleep improves. Even when there are not marked increases in the amount of sleep obtained, this kind of program enables participants to experience a growth of confidence in their ability to cope with sleep disturbance. In one of our studies (M. A. Cook & Lacks, 1984), at the 2-month follow-up, 30% of the clients commented spontaneously that although they still considered themselves to have insomnia, they no longer felt helpless because they now knew concrete and specific ways to deal with their problem. It may be that changes in self-efficacy are subjectively important to insomnia sufferers but are not directly related to reductions in the sleep complaint. Alternatively, changes in self-efficacy may be necessary but not sufficient for improvements in sleep. Regardless, an increase in self-efficacy appears to be a consistent and reliable result of this type of treatment, and its importance has been repeatedly stressed by the participants.

There are many ways in which the behavior therapist can promote an increased sense of self-control. First, we emphasize the active stance that one must take to be successful in this endeavor. A large number of the participants will have previously tried sleep medications and other passive response modes. The behavioral treatment is not a "quick fix."

In fact, we repeatedly invoke counterdemand instructions for clients not to expect any improvement until the fourth week. This is a 4-week program to undo the habits of up to 40 years. Participants cannot expect to change habits in any less than 4 weeks and for some it may take even more time to see substantial improvement. But we are confident that if the client follows the therapy carefully and consistently, the chances are good for developing much-improved sleep. A great deal of emphasis should be placed on the two words *carefully* and *consistently*. Habits are hard to break. You have to force yourself to engage in unnatural patterns of behavior. Any new behavior may often improve a problem for a short time, but we are aiming for a lifestyle change with permanently improved sleep. In many ways this aim is analagous to lifestyle changes in eating patterns and exercise patterns used in weight control, as opposed to the more temporary solution of going on a diet.

Many of our clients have asked us why they could not achieve the same results by just buying and following one of the available self-help books on insomnia (e.g., Coates & Thoresen, 1977). I think one of the reasons that the self-help approach is not particularly successful is that there is no way to control the consistency of practice of the recommended behaviors. Typically, people who try such an approach will follow the instructions erratically over a short time and then conclude that the method does not work. Instead, they have just not given the suggestions a fair chance. Most people appear to need the regular feedback and exhortation provided by a therapist and by other group members to develop the desired active coping skills.

SLEEP HYGIENE AND SLEEP SCHEDULING

Though many individuals know what behaviors and substances can interfere with sleep, they may not necessarily put good sleep hygiene into practice. It is always surprising, but not rare, to find someone who has suffered from sleep disturbance for many years who continues to drink several cups of caffeinated coffee each evening. Practicing poor sleep hygiene may not be the only factor contributing to a person's insomnia; however, as long as there is a physiological basis for sleep disturbance, other attempts to alleviate the problem may fail. Therefore, we take the stance that good sleep hygiene is essential to establish before we move on to other approaches. We always begin the first session by teaching the clients to set up consistently ideal circumstances for sleeping.

One important sleep hygiene issue concerns the withdrawal from sleep-interfering substances such as caffeine. Withdrawal from caffeine can be problematic if the person has been accustomed to ingesting large amounts. Headaches and feelings of anxiety are the most likely caffeine-withdrawal symptoms and can appear after even a brief period of abstinence. Unfortunately, these unpleasant experiences can be reversed by the intake of more caffeine, thus tempting the person to resume the previous levels of consumption. All of these withdrawal patterns are predictable and should be so indicated to the client who is attempting to cut back or to eliminate caffeine intake. It is important that this withdrawal be accomplished before the behavior therapy begins so that withdrawal symptoms are not attributed to the treatment itself. The elimination of exceptionally strong caffeine habits should be supervised by the client's physician. It is interesting that many of our clients who eliminated caffeine usage near bedtime reported that they felt so much better that they decided voluntarily to eliminate caffeine entirely from their lives.

Sleep scheduling is an equally important facet in the overall strategy. Many insomnia sufferers have developed irregular timing of sleep attempts in their efforts to make up for lost sleep at night. Their bodies no longer can count on a naturally occurring sleep rhythm to facilitate sufficient rest at night. Some participants have found that implementing the recommended sleep hygiene and scheduling practices was sufficient to improve their sleep. The specific instructions for this aspect of treatment are detailed in the next chapter.

WITHDRAWAL FROM SLEEP MEDICATION

Before you can begin to provide behavioral treatment for persistent insomnia, it is desirable to have the client withdraw from sleep medications. It is difficult to track the treatment progress of individuals who alter their sleep with drugs. Also, all sleep researchers can cite cases from their experience in which the sole behavior of withdrawal from hypnotics was sufficient to eliminate a person's sleep disturbance. Some clients are eager to rid themselves of this outside influence. Others will be reluctant to do so or may downright refuse. I had one potential research volunteer tell me that she would only forego her hypnotics if I could guarantee the success of the behavioral approach. Of course, the behavioral therapist cannot extend such a warranty. However, because it is well established that sleeping medications can actually cause insomnia and do alter the patterns of sleep as well as result in a variety of side effects, it is in the best interests of the client to give up sleep medications that are taken on a regular and long-term basis.

Most behavior therapists are not physicians and so are not qualified to make this decision. If the client has been taking only an occasional sleeping pill (e.g., no more than once per week), then there should be no medical consequences of eliminating the drugs. If the client has been taking hypnotics more frequently and consistently for some time, it would be dangerous to withdraw abruptly from the drug regimen. A physician will have to plan and supervise a gradual withdrawal program. The most satisfactory arrangement we have developed is for the sleep therapist to fully inform clients who are taking drugs about the dangers and ineffectiveness of this kind of medication. In many cases the sleeping medication only perpetuates the problem it was designed to alleviate. Clients should be warned that during withdrawal they are likely to experience transient rebound insomnia for up to several weeks. We do not want this event to cause them to rush back to their drugs. After providing complete information about drugs, request that clients make an appointment to see the physician who prescribed the pills.

Withdrawal symptoms will vary depending on the dosage and length of usage. Education in these facts ahead of time should help the person to persist with the process of withdrawal. This process may take up to 4 weeks, since many of these drugs have long half-lives. However, as a standard practice, 2 to 3 weeks is probably sufficient time for most individuals. With drugs of short half-life, withdrawal symptoms usually appear right away, whereas with drugs of longer half-life, such as the benzodiazepines, problems may not appear for up to a week (American Medical Association, 1984).

The physician should work out a timetable of regular and gradual reduction of the drugs with amounts being lowered once or twice a week. A good deal of support and patience from the therapist and from the physician will be called for during this period, as well as reminders that the client is engaging in a health-promoting activity that will eventually improve sleep. Discussions of the rewards that will ensue from the client's future feelings of self-efficacy may also be helpful (VanOot et al., 1984). These comments about withdrawal from sleep medications are also applicable to elimination of alcohol as a sleep aid as long as the person cannot be classified as alcoholic. In the latter case, referral to Alcoholics Anonymous or another chemical dependency treatment program may be necessary. Therapy for insomnia in these clients may need to await a later date or be done on an individual basis rather than within a group of people who have only sleeping problems.

Kirmil-Gray, Eagleston, Thoresen, and Zarcone (1985) have published one of the few empirical reports of withdrawal from sleeping medication. They assigned 6 drug-dependent women to a brief individual consultation program that included structure, support, and health education. Another 6 women received a more extensive group-administered stress management therapy that taught relaxation and cognitive skills. These women had used drugs or alcohol to promote sleep for an average of 10 years, most of them 7 nights a week. After stabilizing the drug usage, reductions were made at the rate of about one clinical dose every 1 to 2 weeks. The women in the consultation program received an average of about 2 hours of group orientation and 3 hours of individual contact time; those in the stress management condition received 24 hours of group time. All 12 subjects succeeded in withdrawing totally from sleep medication within a median time of 6.5 weeks. Sleep without medication did not deteriorate but rather improved slightly on several EEG measures. Those in the stress management group made greater improvements than did those in the consultation group. At a 6-month follow-up, none of the women had returned to nightly use of hypnotics. Half were using medication no more than 2 times per month and the other half 1 to 4 times per week.

These researchers recommend the following key elements for a sleep-medication withdrawal program: (a) a written plan of the withdrawal schedule, (b) sleep hygiene information to promote better sleep during this period, (c) regular brief appointments and phone calls to hold the client accountable for reduction of medication and to check on progress, (d) consistent support and encouragement from the health professional, and (e) daily monitoring on diaries of sleep and medication use.

Ideally, the client would be drug-free for a period of 2 to 4 weeks before even beginning baseline sleep diaries. Although the client may be impatient to begin therapy, it is wise to reiterate that the insomnia is longstanding and that it will not be intolerable to wait a few more weeks before obtaining relief. Our research team has been committed to providing drug-free treatment for persistent insomnia. In line with this philosophy we have not accepted for therapy anyone who was unwilling to discontinue sleep medication. However, some clinicians may be willing to experiment with weaning clients from their drugs gradually while they participate in therapy. If such a course is followed, it is likely that treatment will need to be lengthened beyond the usual 4 weeks. Turner and Ascher (1979) allowed clients to continue drug use during treatment and found that mean weekly drug usage did drop from the baseline figure of about 4 nights (across 3 treatments); however, at posttreatment clients were still using drugs about 2.5 nights per week.

PREPARING FOR EACH SESSION

The therapist will have to be well organized if the considerable goals of the first session are going to be achieved in 60 to 90 minutes. Generally the last 3 sessions only require an hour each. For each session you will want to have the following materials:

- Decaffeinated coffee
- Name tags and markers
- Treatment instruction sheets
- Sleep diaries
- Daily homework logs
- Specific questionnaires
- Pencils
- Folders for each client to store handouts
- List of participants' names

As people assemble for the initial meeting, you might ask the first person who arrives to take charge of distributing name tags. Ask that clients only use first names to preserve some degree of confidentiality.

Chapter 7
The First Treatment Session

BREAKING THE ICE

The first order of business is for the therapist to introduce himself or herself and, if appropriate, to say a few words about personal background or experience in the treatment of insomnia. The therapist may want to mention any personally experienced previous sleep difficulties that have since been resolved. A short description of the research findings in the treatment of sleep problems may also be desirable. The object of this brief beginning is to get group members to relax, to promote their feeling of confidence in the therapist, and to arouse an expectation of success.

Next, the therapist should have the group members introduce themselves and describe briefly their own histories of insomnia in terms of how long it has been a problem, how frequently they experience these problems, how severe they perceive their problem to be, what solutions they have already tried, and what their current motivation is to seek help for this problem. This process is a way to break the ice and make clients more comfortable with each other. Many insomnia sufferers perceive having a sleep disorder as a stigma. Hearing other essentially normal people describe problems so similar to their own comes as a major relief to them. As each person finishes, the therapist should try to emphasize the similarities among the problems that have been described, especially any that fit into the rationale of the treatment that will be offered (e.g., performance anxiety, disrupted sleep scheduling, worrying in bed). Also during this segment, begin to foster a group interaction. For example, after each person speaks, you might ask the other group members to comment or to ask questions about what has just been said. Allow about 10 to 15 minutes for this segment.

THE CONCEPT OF STIMULUS CONTROL

It is important that all of the following information be communicated to the group. However, the therapist needs to learn the material thoroughly so that it can be presented in an informal way, rather than giving a droning lecture or even reading it verbatim. Most of the participants will not be familiar with the concept of stimulus control although they can readily understand it if presented in terms of their everyday experiences.

Much of what we do is influenced by the time and the place we are in. The *stimulus*, or characteristic of a situation, gets paired with the behavior that occurs in that situation. The characteristics of the situation then become a signal or *cue* for that behavior.

There are many examples from your everyday life of this phenomenon. For example, did any of you ever eat a large meal, feel entirely satisfied, and then go to a movie? What experience did you have when you entered the lobby of the theater? Many of you probably wanted a box of popcorn and a soda (or candy etc.) even though you knew that you were not in the least hungry! Through years of experience of having popcorn most of the times that you went to the movies, the lobby of the theater has come to be a strong cue for you to want popcorn. The stimulus *controls*, or *cues*, the behavior. Other common examples are feeling hungry when the clock says noon even if you ate only 2 hours before; wanting a cigarette after each meal or with each cup of coffee; feeling alarmed when the phone rings in the middle of the night, but not experiencing any anxiety when the phone rings during the day.

See if group members can come up with their own examples.

For people who sleep well, the bed and bedroom act as a signal to feel sleepy and to fall asleep quickly. You may hear these people complain that each time they put their head on the pillow they fall asleep immediately even when they had intentions to read for a while. It may have been very hard for you to feel much sympathy for their dilemma. For people who have insomnia, the bed and bedroom may have become a signal for other activities. These activities include lying awake, thinking and worrying, feeling frustrated about not sleeping, reading, watching television, and other similar behaviors.

Sometimes this connection begins after something happens that disrupts normal sleep. For example, a stressful event such as divorce, a change in your job, or a new baby may have this effect.

See if any clients connect the beginning of their insomnia with a specific event and encourage discussion on this point.

After the disruption or stress is over, poor sleep, frustration, and any activities that the poor sleeper may have performed while waiting for sleep (e.g., reading, watching television) remain associated with the bed and bedroom. Subsequently, the bed remains a cue for these nonsleeping behaviors and for being awake. The occasional nights of poor sleep that everyone experiences reinforce these connections.

BRIEF DESCRIPTION OF BEHAVIORAL TREATMENT FOR INSOMNIA

At this point, explain that you are going to describe briefly the treatment but that they should not worry if they do not fully understand it right away. Shortly, you will be handing out written instructions, which you will go over point by point. For now, they should not worry about the details but instead should just try to get a feel for what will be implemented.

In this treatment, we will be using a multifaceted behavior therapy approach to a complicated problem. Included will be education about sleep, sleep monitoring, and a procedure called stimulus control. The stimulus control approach was developed by Dr. Richard Bootzin at Northwestern University and has been widely researched across the country.

With stimulus control you will learn to reassociate the bed and bedroom with rapid sleep onset. The bed and bedroom will be weakened as a cue for other activities. You will learn to maximize the cues that are associated with feeling sleepy and falling asleep, and to decrease the cues that are associated with staying awake.

In addition to using these stimulus control procedures, you will learn to acquire a consistent sleep rhythm through sleep scheduling. You will also learn which behaviors and substances (such as caffeine) interfere with sleep, and how to eliminate or reschedule them.

You will be developing new, permanent sleep habits. I will not be doing anything *to* you. I will be helping you discover old habits and cues that are keeping you awake. Then I will be helping you to develop new habits that will help you fall asleep rapidly and stay asleep.

For this therapy to work, you will have to monitor your behavior carefully. You will also have to practice the recommended new behaviors consistently so that they become routine or habitual. Even after you are sleeping better, you must continue to use the new habits regularly.

Make an analogy to new eating habits for weight control or to reduction of salt intake to control high blood pressure.

Once you have learned these new behaviors, you will use them consistently every day to ensure that they become habits. Are there any questions?

Make sure clients buy this explanation of insomnia and why this treatment works. Clarify any issues or uncertainties raised by group members.

INSERTING THE COUNTERDEMAND

Insert the following instructions in a spontaneous way and repeat throughout the sessions as necessary.

We estimate that after the fourth session you will begin to experience dramatic improvement. However, during the first 3 weeks, we do not expect much improvement, so do not get discouraged. In fact, after this first week of practicing my recommendations, you will probably feel *worse* for a few days. It is only after 4 sessions and careful practice on your own that the real improvement will occur.

NINE SLEEP HYGIENE RULES

At this point you will introduce the group to the sleep hygiene element of their therapy. Begin by handing out a written copy of the rules. You may prepare your own or use those printed in Table 7.1. It is best to present this list separately from other instructions to prevent members from jumping ahead of you. First, let the group members briefly read the list. Then go over each point on the list, providing further explanation. For each point:

1. Read the rule.
2. Elaborate the rule.
3. Have each client discuss their current behavior in relation to the rule.
4. Have each client discuss implementing the rule, including *concrete strategies* for using it in their life.

When appropriate, record the planned new behaviors to serve as a reference in future sessions.

Rule 1: Lie down with the intention of going to sleep *only* when you feel drowsy and ready for sleep.
    Many insomnia sufferers go to bed before they are sleepy. If they had a hard time getting to sleep the night before, they probably feel tired and they reason that they should get an earlier start on their sleep tonight. Sometimes these people spend 10 to 12 hours in bed trying to get 8 hours of sleep. Let your body tell you when it is drowsy. If you go to bed when you are sleepy, you are more likely to go to sleep right away, reinforcing

Table 7.1. Sleep Hygiene Rules

---

1. Do not go to bed until you are drowsy.
2. Get up at approximately the same time each morning, including weekends. If you feel you must get up later on weekends, allow yourself a maximum of 1 hour later arising.
3. Do not take naps.

These first 3 rules will give you a consistent sleep rhythm and synchronize your biological clock. With time, your bedtime, or the time you become drowsy, will also tend to become regularized.

4. Do not drink alcohol later than 2 hours prior to bedtime.
5. Do not consume caffeine after about 4 p.m., or within 6 hours prior to bedtime. Learn all the foods, beverages, and medications that contain caffeine.
6. Do not smoke within several hours prior to your bedtime.
7. Exercise regularly. The best time to exercise is in the late afternoon. Avoid strenuous physical exertion after 6 p.m.
8. Use common sense to make your sleep environment most conducive to sleep. Arrange for a comfortable temperature and minimum levels of sound, light, and noise.
9. If you are accustomed to it, have a light carbohydrate snack before bedtime (e.g., crackers, graham crackers, milk, or cheese). Do not eat chocolate or large amounts of sugar. Avoid excessive fluids. If you awaken in the middle of the night, do not have a snack then or you may find that you begin to wake up habitually at that time feeling hungry.

---

the association between bed and sleep. If you are not sleepy, you might toss and turn, begin to think, and get mentally and physically aroused. That would only reinforce the old habit patterns we are trying to eliminate. Remember, being tired does not necessarily mean you are drowsy or ready for sleep.

Some people worry that they will not get enough sleep if they follow this rule because the time they have to get up cannot change, due to work and schedule demands. But, by establishing a fixed time for getting up and allowing your bedtime to vary, your body can determine how much sleep you actually do need in order to function well. Eventually your body will send you this message by getting sleepy when it is time for you to go to bed.

Discuss how clients are now determining when they will go to bed (e.g., a fixed versus flexible bedtime or one that is linked to the spouse's bedtime). Ask how sleepy or awake they feel when they go to bed. Determine how clients can tell when they feel sleepy (e.g., yawning, rubbing eyes, flickering eyelids). It is amazing how many insomniacs think that they have no way of knowing when they are drowsy. Many have to be taught concretely how to recognize the cues of drowsiness. Tell clients that these cues will be a little different for each of them. Have each person become more aware of his or her own feelings and signs of sleepiness and tell clients to use these feelings as a cue to go to bed.

Rule 2: Get up at the same time every morning regardless of how much sleep you got during the night or how rested you feel. Use an alarm clock to make sure that you accomplish this consistent wake-up time. It is important to permit your body to establish a regular body rhythm of peaks and lows. Sleeping in late on some mornings will accomplish much the same kind of effect that traveling across time zones does to your sleep patterns. Many poor sleepers use weekend mornings for trying to recapture some of the sleep they lost during the week. We will firmly discourage this practice because it only exacerbates problems with sleep. If you sleep in on weekend mornings you will not be ready to fall asleep at your usual time at night, setting the stage for insomnia for the rest of the week. If you feel that getting up at the same time on weekends is a special hardship for you, let's talk about it. I want you to try to follow this rule during the 4 weeks of treatment. If you continue to feel strongly about this point, once the active phase of the therapy has been completed you can allow yourself up to a maximum of 1 hour later arising on Saturday and Sunday. Follow this same weekend rule for vacation days.

Discuss when clients now get up. How do they determine when they will get up? What means do they use to wake up? How consistent are their awakening times, including weekends? Have each client set a time to get up every morning. Explore how well the client can live with the time, and change it if necessary. Record these waking-up times. You can set up the list of clients' names in such a way that you can also record this type of information. If you prefer, you can develop a specific form for this purpose. Whatever the format, the therapist will need to keep careful records of planned behaviors and individualized home-work assignments in order to check on progress in subsequent sessions.

Rule 3: Do not take daytime naps. Most sleep experts are convinced that napping almost always disrupts the sleep arousal rhythm, making it harder to sleep at night. One reason for this disruption is that most people who do take naps do so some days but not others and take their naps at varying times each day. If you take naps you may also interfere with your body's natural ability to get the needed combination of all the different stages of sleep.

These procedures described in the first 3 instructions will help your body to acquire a consistent sleep rhythm so that you feel drowsy and ready for sleep at about the same time each night and feel alert and ready to awaken at about the same time each morning.

Discuss with clients whether they now have a habit of taking naps and how often they do so. Find out if it will be difficult for them to give up these naps. Discuss other activities they might substitute for a nap when they are feeling daytime drowsiness. Examples might include an afternoon walk, jog, or swim. If a client insists on taking naps, the naps should not exceed an hour and should be taken regularly and at approximately the same time each day.

Before elaborating the next 3 instructions, you should discuss briefly how insomnia can result from a disruption of our natural sleep cycles by lifestyle factors or by bad habits we have acquired. These lifestyle factors and habits are called sleep hygiene. Describe briefly how most of us are born good sleepers and that this natural ability becomes disrupted by lifestyle habits we acquire as we become adults. An example might be the person who drinks many cups of coffee throughout the day and evening or the health-conscious individual who exercises during the hour just prior to bedtime to get worn out as an inducement to sleep. Both of these activities are likely to make sleep more difficult. By changing these habits, clients may allow their bodies to reestablish the natural tendency to be a good sleeper. These new practices alone may not be sufficient to eliminate the sleep difficulty; however, they will set the stage for the other treatment procedures to work. If a person followed every action recommended in this treatment but still drank coffee at night, he or she might still continue to experience insomnia.

Rule 4: Do not drink alcohol later than 2 hours prior to bedtime. Although alcohol is a depressant, which if timed accurately may aid you to relax and fall asleep, it leads to restless, nonrestorative sleep and the tendency to wake up during the night.

Rule 5: Do not drink caffeine later than 6 hours before bedtime. Caffeine is a powerful and long-lasting stimulant that interferes with the natural sleep cycle.

Spend a brief amount of time educating the group as to which substances contain caffeine and in what amounts. Myths abound in this area. For example, many people believe that tea has far less caffeine than coffee although they actually have equivalent amounts. Use the information presented in chapter 2 to acquaint the group with the presence of caffeine. Some medications contain caffeine or other stimulants so be sure to explore any prescribed drugs they may be using. We teach our clients the importance of checking labels and of talking with their physicians or pharmacists about alternative medications that do not contain stimulants. The physician may also be able to recommend a different schedule for taking the medication, such as earlier in the day and not in the evening. Strongly discourage any client from eliminating a prescribed medication without consulting the physician.

Rule 6: If you smoke, try not to smoke within several hours of your bedtime. Like caffeine, nicotine is a powerful stimulant.

After each of the preceding 3 instructions, discuss clients' current patterns in regard to that activity. Reinforce any comments that are compatible with the rationale provided for avoiding these 3 activities near bedtime. Determine if there will be any compliance problems and have the group make suggestions. These 3 instructions often elicit a good deal of resistance because many such habits are strongly entrenched. Clients will insist that they already follow these rules or that they tried them before with no success. Do not accept this excuse. Careful questioning about what they tried and how often will usually reveal that they only partially followed the rules or did so for a short time or inconsistently. Someone may have given up coffee at night but still eats chocolate or mocha ice cream before retiring. Some clients will think that these rules are simplistic and silly. Others will feel a tremendous sense of deprivation at having to give up these substances. Many of them use stimulants to help alleviate the symptoms of fatigue from sleeplessness. Though quite a few group members may be familiar with the interfering effects of these substances upon sleep, they do not avoid them and only give lip service to the necessity to do so.

Rule 7: Do not have vigorous exercise immediately prior to bedtime. Exercise stimulates the body and makes falling asleep soon afterward very difficult. Exercise just before bed does not tire us out but has the paradoxical effect of waking us up. In fact, people who are drowsy and trying to stay awake to study often engage in physical exercise to wake themselves up. However, exercise in the late afternoon or early evening is a worthwhile pursuit and can be a good substitute for caffeine to ward off early evening drowsiness.

Rule 8: Set up your sleeping environment to make it conducive to sleep. Discuss light, temperature, mattresses, noise levels, and other relevant factors. A white noise machine can mask outside noises (e.g., Sleep Mate II available through the Sears catalogue). Many people also find this steady sound to be soothing and sleep inducing.

Rule 9: If you are accustomed to it, you may have a light carbohydrate snack before bedtime.

If a poor sleeper does not currently eat a bedtime snack and does not complain of sleeplessness due to hunger, there is no reason to start having a nighttime snack. However, if the client is already eating such a snack and considers it important to do so, he or she may continue this practice. You may want to discuss what is being eaten and in what amounts to make sure that it is an appropriate snack. It is important, however, that no one eat a snack in the middle of the night or they may train themselves to wake up at that time to eat. If someone reports consistently waking up hungry in the night, that person should experiment with a prebedtime snack. Chocolate and excessive amounts of sugar can serve as stimulants. A large fluid intake in the evening is likely to cause nighttime awakenings to urinate.

STIMULUS CONTROL INSTRUCTIONS

Now pass out the separate sheet of directions for this part of the treatment. You may make up your own handout or you may make copies of Table 7.2.

Instruction 1: Do not use your bed or bedroom for any activity other than sleep. You should not read, watch television, talk on the telephone, eat, argue with your spouse, or worry in bed. Sexual activity is the only exception to this rule. If you do engage in sexual activity and do not feel sleepy afterwards, do not use the bed for other activities at that time. Doing other things in bed is "misusing" the bed. There is an appropriate time and place for everything. Doing other things reinforces the notion that a variety of actions are appropriate in that setting. For example, if you often watch television in bed, going to bed can become a cue to want to watch television or to begin thinking about things you have seen on television. If the bed is reserved for sleep alone, then climbing into bed will be a strong cue for you to fall asleep.

Have clients discuss other activities they currently carry out in bed. Be sure to include thinking, worrying, feeling frustrated about not falling asleep, important discussions, and arguments with their spouse.

Table 7.2. Stimulus Control Instructions

1. Do not use your bed or bedroom for any activity other than sleep. You should not watch television, read, talk on the telephone, worry, argue with your spouse, or eat in bed. The only exception to this rule is that you may engage in sexual activity in bed.
2. Establish a set of regular presleep routines to signal that bedtime approaches. Lock the door, plug in the coffee machine, brush teeth, set the alarm, and perform any other behaviors that make sense for this time of night. Do these activities in the same order each night. Use your preferred sleep posture and combination of favorite pillows and blankets.
3. When you get into bed, turn out the lights with the intention of going right to sleep. If you cannot fall asleep within a short time (about 10 minutes), get up and go into another room. Engage in some quiet activity until you begin to feel drowsy and then return to the bedroom to sleep.
4. If you still do not fall asleep within a brief time, repeat the previous step. Repeat this process as often as it is necessary throughout the night. Use this same procedure if you awaken in the middle of the night and do not return to sleep within about 10 minutes.

Restate that there is an appropriate time and place for everything. Discourage clients from trying to give up these other activities. If they are doing them, they must be enjoyable or important to the client and should not be given up. Discuss other times and places to carry out these activities. For example, time can be set aside earlier in the evening to have a discussion with a spouse in the living room. One can also select a half hour before or after dinner to review in one's mind the events of the day and to plan the upcoming one. Get concrete solutions to carrying out these activities in places other than the bed and bedroom. These solutions often include moving things such as television sets and desks out of the bedroom. The therapist should jot down these plans for reference during future sessions.

Instruction 2: Establish a set of regular presleep routines that signal the approach of bedtime. The hour before bedtime should be one during which you prepare for sleep, a time to wind down. Presleep activities often include some kind of relaxation, a putting aside of the troubles of the day just past and of the day to come. Typical ways to relax at this time are to take a warm bath, to read, or to watch television. It is not relaxing to begin a new project, to start an argument with a spouse, to go for a 3-mile jog, make an important business call, or plan the business agenda for the following day. Those kinds of things should be scheduled for earlier in the day. Many good sleepers have a regular group of prebedtime activities — such as locking the door, brushing their teeth, setting the alarm — that they carry out consistently. Engaging in this routine is one of the beginning cues that it is time to go to sleep. This topic will be covered in more detail in the second session.

Instruction 3: When you get into bed, turn out the lights with the intention of going right to sleep. If you find that you cannot fall asleep within a short time, get up and go into another room. Stay up as long as it takes until you begin to feel drowsy, and then return to the bedroom to sleep. Although I do not want you to be a clockwatcher, I want you to get out of bed if you do not fall asleep fairly soon. Remember, your goal is to come to associate your bed with falling asleep *quickly*! Use a period of about 10 minutes as your guideline. If you are in bed awake more than this amount of time and have not gotten out of bed, you are not following the treatment.

Return to bed only when you feel sleepy. The object is for you to connect the bed and bedroom with sleeping. Often, the bed originally became a cue for other activities because the poor sleeper would watch television, eat, read, and engage in other activities as a distraction from the primary concern — not falling asleep. With time, however, because of this lengthy association of the bed with these activities, it has become a signal to engage in these other behaviors whenever in bed.

If you stay in bed, the bed also becomes a cue for worrying about insomnia and all the anxiety and frustration over not falling asleep. As a result, the insomnia sufferer comes to fight the bed. Some poor sleepers even refer to their bed and bedroom as the *enemy*. This process is the reason some people who suffer from insomnia fall asleep better in places other than their own beds, for example in a chair while watching television or in a hotel or even in a sleep laboratory with wires glued to their head. Good sleepers show just the opposite pattern — they have more difficulty falling asleep outside of their own bed.

See if any clients have the experience of falling asleep easily outside of their own bed. Discuss with clients what they do now when they cannot fall asleep. Elicit concrete examples. Discuss where they will go and what they will do when they cannot fall asleep. Begin with the activities they are doing now, such as reading, and help them find another place to do it. Encourage clients who are already following this rule to some extent. Shape their behavior to conform to the rule more completely and consistently. *Do not* continue with the session until each client has some concrete alternatives for what to do if he or she does not fall asleep right away. Record these strategies for each client.

Help clients plan what activities they will engage in outside of the bedroom when they get up. For example, some may decide that they will read. They should know what they will need to prepare for this activity — the book or magazine, reading glasses, a small flashlight (or a nightlight), and a robe set aside in a convenient place so they do not disturb their bedpartner when they get up.

Instruction 4: If you still have not fallen asleep, repeat the previous step. Repeat this process as often as it is necessary throughout the night. The new habits will come only with repeated practice. When you begin this treatment, it is common to have to get up many times each night before falling asleep. In fact, when you return next week, many of you will probably feel that your insomnia is worse than when you began therapy for it. We frequently hear people say at the second session that the cure is worse than the problem they came with. Do not despair. After this first week you will not have to be getting out of bed so often. Also, you will probably not be losing any more sleep than you did before; it will just seem like it. To prove my prediction, I am going to have you keep track of how many times you get up each night and bring this record with you to each session. Although this instruction may be the single most difficult one for you to comply with in the treatment, it is probably also the single most important one for you to follow.

Impress upon the group members that it takes good sleepers from 5 to 10 minutes to fall asleep. Group members should also use this getting-out-of-bed procedure any time that they wake up in the middle of the night. Discuss what they do now if they wake up during the night. Briefly discuss repeatedly using the strategies that they developed under instruction 3. Clients should now be told to begin following all of these rules tonight.

It is important that you reemphasize how difficult it will be for them to follow these rules at first. Initial difficulty is typical for any new behavior a person is trying to incorporate. Clients should expect their sleep to get worse the first week. They will not want to comply with the instructions as they realize it is difficult and seems to be making their sleep go downhill. Predict for them these immediate negative consequences.

For the first few nights you will be getting up many times before falling asleep; you will get little sleep, and you will feel tired and have impaired functioning during the day. During these first few days you will probably feel quite discouraged and may even consider dropping out of the treatment program. But for most people this worsening of the target behavior is temporary, a few nights or a week at most. After that you should see a leveling-off effect and then a gradual improvement. The temporary negative consequences are the inevitable result of breaking old habits and of establishing a consistent sleep rhythm when there was none before.

PRETREATMENT EXPECTATIONS

Somewhere near the end of the first session, you may want to have clients indicate their initial reactions to the description of the treatment being offered. We ask clients to rate on 7-point scales how logical the treatment seems, how confident they are it will be successful, and how confident they would be in recommending it to a friend with insomnia (Borkovec & Nau, 1972). You will probably get a more honest response if you ask the clients not to put their names on these evaluations. By reviewing client reactions to this first session, the therapist can gain some feedback on how well the presentation has gone and how it has influenced the client's expectations. Ask the group to fill out the form as candidly as possible.

During the explanation of the rationale and the description of the therapy, it will be important that the group members come to accept the therapist and buy into the rationale. In our research, we have found uniformly high ratings on these 3 questions. If you find that you obtain lower ratings, you may want to examine your style as well as the content of your presentation, or have a colleague give you feedback. Although the group members will typically indicate in writing that they have high expectations for what you have described, you can also expect some verbal resistance in the group discussion. It is not uncommon for one or more participants to report that they have already tried this therapy or some parts of it. With further exploration, you will usually find that they did only some part of it, usually for a very brief time, and rarely with any consistency.

With that information, you can restate your strongly held conviction that it will take 4 weeks of careful and consistent practice for these instructions to have a beneficial effect. Also state that some of the instructions may seem simplistic, silly, or unnecessary. However, each part of this treatment package is derived from a good deal of research with a large number of insomnia sufferers. Each part is designed to contribute to the final positive result. If the clients tamper with the overall plan, picking and choosing only those elements that they want, they will seriously compromise their chances of improving their sleep. We insist that they really have nothing to lose by cooperating fully. They have suffered for a long time now or they would not be here. They have gone to a lot of trouble and expense to end up in this group. We are asking them to do *possible* things for a very short period of time. So for 4 weeks, doesn't it make the most sense to go ahead and give it their best try? Once you have a sense of which group members have bought the rationale and are willing to give it a try, use them to bring peer pressure on those who are expressing doubts.

ASSIGNING HOMEWORK

Repeat the importance of following the sleep hygiene and stimulus control instructions every day. Explain that an important part of building new, better sleep habits is monitoring sleep-related behaviors closely to identify and strengthen which cues are associated with falling asleep quickly. The clients also need to identify and weaken those cues associated with staying awake. Thus, throughout treatment clients will be closely monitoring and charting their sleep-related behaviors.

Explain in detail the sheets titled Practice Record and Number of Times Out of Bed (see Appendix). Include instructions on how to fill out the 6 questions and how to chart the number of times they had to get up each night before falling asleep. Explain that in each future session, a good deal of time will be spent going over the practice records, so it is important that each client fill out these records faithfully and bring them to all sessions. Hand out 7 new stamped diaries and reemphasize the crucial importance of filling these out each morning upon awakening and mailing them in each day. Describe briefly what will happen in future sessions. Ask for questions and comments. Make sure each group member understands the homework assignment.

The end of the session is also a good time to emphasize the importance of the upcoming meetings, and to point out that 4 weeks of treatment is not very long and that their attendance at all meetings will be necessary for the maximum benefit. Announce the dates and times of all the sessions and find out if there will be time conflicts for any member. If possible, arrange to have persons with such conflicts attend the same session in another ongoing group or else have them come in for a 15-minute individual session to cover the important material. Arrange to give extra diaries to anyone who will be going out of town.

Chapter 8
Subsequent Sessions

The majority of the next 3 sessions will be spent in a collaborative troubleshooting of any problems that group members have encountered in adhering to the treatment during the week. Although some new material is introduced in each of these 3 sessions, the problem solving will take up most of the time. We have developed a standard format to use for this problem solving. The following procedures should be used to discuss any difficulties that arise as clients attempt to carry out the rules of the therapy.

FORMAT FOR PROBLEM SOLVING

1. Use the practice records to elicit any problems with adherence to treatment.

Before the session begins, as the clients trickle in, collect and review briefly the homework or practice record forms. Doing this will allow you to be somewhat prepared for the general content that might be brought up during group discussions. Knowing what the actual data are will also help you to combat effectively any tendency for a client to exaggerate negatively what really happened during the week. Clients can use this time before the formal meeting starts to talk among themselves and get to know each other better. Return the forms to the clients and use the first part of each of sessions 2, 3, and 4 to address systematically each of the 6 homework questions. Take up each question separately and go around the group asking all members to report what experiences and problems they had. At the end of the session, collect and keep these forms for future reference and planning.

2. Get a full description of the problem.

If clients report having encountered difficulties during the week, ask each person to describe the problem. Have them each be as precise as possible. Try to determine if the problem was the client's inability or unwillingness to carry out the procedures or if it was the environment that made it difficult for the client to follow the rules. Ask clients to explain how they formulate the problem, what they see as the difficulty. If the problem seems inconsequential, let the client know that it will have little effect on the ability to gain better sleep habits and that there is no need to continue to worry about it.

3. Try for a group problem solving process as much as is possible.

Let the client and the group come up with possible solutions for each problem. Encourage discussion and a sharing of experiences. What worked for other clients in similar situations? At first generate as many solutions as possible without any criticisms. After this brainstorming, combine and improve suggestions. Make the solutions as specific as possible.

4. Maintain a committment to the stimulus control approach to treatment of insomnia.

Strongly emphasize the importance of following the rules every night. Do not tolerate clients' breaking the treatment rules or not carrying out the behaviors they agreed to do. Remind clients of the rationale behind stimulus control and why it is an effective treatment for insomnia.

5. Decide upon a course of action for the coming week.

Choose the solution that has the most useful consequences and that the client seems most likely to implement. Maintain an air of confidence. Communicate to the client that problems are routine and solvable and any particular difficulty is neither unique nor insurmountable. Predict what the likely consequences will be including any possible side effects.

6.   Have the client try the behavior during the week.

Stress the "personal scientist" strategy of problem solving. Once a potential solution is identified, that course of action can be implemented with a trial and error philosophy. The behavior is being tried conditionally pending its outcome. If it does not work, one simply decides on another potential solution. During the experiments, clients should monitor the success of the new behavior so that they can report back to the group the following week.

7.   Defer a problem solution if necessary.

If the group or the therapist cannot come up with a solution immediately, have the client carefully monitor the problem and behavior connected with it for the next week. Present this as a routine way to find solutions. Do not communicate the message that the therapist has never faced this problem before. During the week, devise a solution. If the problem still exists the following week, present the proposed solution to the client.

8.   Always follow up on progress.

Be sure to pursue problems discussed the week before and how well the solutions worked. This therapist behavior conveys the attitude that you are always monitoring client progress and that you take adherence to treatment seriously. Do not tolerate clients' not employing suggestions. Find new solutions if necessary.

9.   Restate the counterdemand.

Remind clients that they are learning new habits and that these behaviors must be practiced consistently over at least the 4-week treatment period to work and to become routine. Treat all reports of progress with surprise and respond to expressed lack of change with encouragement and patience. Individualize success by saying something like, "Well it's great that the treatment is working for you, but most permanent changes don't begin to occur until the procedures have been followed for at least 3 weeks." This approach prevents those clients who have not yet succeeded from becoming discouraged.

10.   Reinforce progress.

Point out any improvements in the clients' ability to follow the rules and new routines. Give plenty of praise and encouragement. Use the group members to praise and support each other.

SESSION 2

Expect the second session to be the hardest. Many of the clients are going to feel frustrated and discouraged; some may even be angry that their symptoms and distress got worse during this week. Your position should be that you warned them that this worsening would take place. If their sleep did deteriorate during the past week, then they were following the treatment instructions. This worsening means that they are right on track and the treatment is taking its expected course.

One topic that almost always surfaces in this second session is the extreme aversion clients have toward getting out of bed after a brief period of sleeplessness. They find all kinds of reasons why they do not want to leave the comfort of their warm bed, especially in the winter months. As much as you may be tempted to modify this requirement, do not do it! This instruction is essential to the success of the program. Instead, focus your efforts and those of the group on ways to make the task less aversive. Preparation ahead of time of all the materials needed to get out of bed and go to another room does a lot to facilitate the behavior. Contrast the immediate discomfort of leaving the bed with the long-term gains of improved sleep. In the near future, with better sleep, there will no longer be a need to get out of bed. Usually there will be at least one group member who has faithfully complied with this requirement and is already starting to notice some alleviation of the sleep problem. Use this person as an example and encourage him or her to coach the others.

Another frequent excuse for not getting out of bed is that it might disturb the bedpartner. When more details are gained, it often turns out that the partner has never complained about being disturbed or may not even be aware that the poor sleeper has left the bed. Because chronic insomniacs have so much performance anxiety about their own sleep being disturbed, they often attribute the same concerns to good sleepers. Just as often, worry about disturbing someone else serves as a convenient excuse not to engage in a difficult behavior.

Encourage the client to discuss the matter with the bedpartner. Find out exactly what behaviors the partner would object to or would find disturbing. Do not allow the client to assume what the partner is thinking without checking it out. Most likely the bedpartner is willing to endure a bit of inconvenience temporarily if it will lead to improvements in the client's sleep. It is unlikely that the noise and movement of the client's leaving the bed are any more disturbing than that of the client's tossing and turning while awake in bed. Some spouses may sabotage treatment, but more often they do not know how to be supportive of the insomniac. Encourage clients to tell their family what their needs are and to solicit their support.

Another difficulty that will be reported by a number of group members is adherence to sleep hygiene rules. Giving up certain substances or practices after many years can result in strong feelings of deprivation. These clients will require a lot of support and encouragement from the therapist and other group members. The importance of good sleep hygiene in eliminating insomnia should be reiterated and methods of active problem solving promoted.

Other topics that usually come up in the second session are questions about what kinds of activities are appropriate when waiting to become drowsy, what cues help you know when you are drowsy, and how you estimate when a period of 10 minutes has passed. The choice of activities for the period before bedtime or when the poor sleeper has left the bed is an important issue. The point is to avoid any activity that promotes alertness. Some examples of inappropriate choices are starting on the last 50 pages of a book the client has been reading, reading an engrossing thriller novel, watching a television movie and wanting to see how it ends, or doing work brought home from the office. The ideal passtime will be something that can just as readily be discontinued after 2 minutes, 15 minutes, or 2 hours, whenever the client gets sleepy. Most clients choose to read either something very boring or a magazine with brief articles, or to watch the equivalent on television, such as a late-night variety show. They should not engage in anything that will stimulate them to think or ruminate. Be sure to review with each person what to do during sleepless periods in order to make sure that it is an appropriate choice.

Some poor sleepers insist that, "I never get sleepy." We suspect that they are confusing the words *sleepy* and *drowsy*. Cues to drowsiness for most people are yawning, eyelids feeling heavy, eyes rolling back, reading the same line several times and not understanding it, having minilapses of attention while watching television, and the head drooping. Some people may have more idiosyncratic responses, such as eyes watering or difficulty maintaining visual focus while reading. Generally, a brief discussion of these signs suffices to clarify the cues of readiness for sleep.

Because many poor sleepers tend to have an obsessive quality to their personality, it is not unusual to have clients ask for guidance in being able to determine when *exactly* 10 minutes of sleeplessness have passed. Some have very creative suggestions, like a clock that projects the time on the bedroom ceiling. I heard a report of one woman who had clocks scattered all over her bedroom so that whatever position she took in her bed she could see what time it was. The therapist should deemphasize the use of clocks in general. Clockwatching only leads to performance anxiety. Whenever clients have been in bed for a short time and they feel they have lost their sense of drowsiness, they should get out of bed. It is not so important that they wait for the whole 10 minutes. Much more important is that they do not lie there too long and begin to ruminate, feel anxious, or have racing thoughts. Because of their years of practice insomniacs tend to be rather accurate estimators of the passage of time. One suggestion is that during the day they can practice estimating a 10-minute period using a kitchen timer.

Establishing a Prebed Routine

The designated new material for Session 2 concerns the establishment of a set of prebed routines. Just as the bed and bedroom can become cues for feeling sleepy and falling asleep quickly, prebed activities can also be a cue to feel sleepy, once a bedtime routine has been established. Some good sleepers report that just getting ready for bed is enough to make them feel more sleepy. Research has shown that children who assume the same particular posture when going to bed fall asleep faster.

Have your clients look over their responses to the Practice Record question concerning activities while getting ready for bed. Ask them to look for patterns of behaviors they always or usually performed. What was the order in which the activities were carried out? How consistent or varied are their presleep routines now? Discuss how sleepy they felt when they began to get ready for bed.

Use their current activities and whatever pattern they found as a starting point to develop a routine. Have clients list the behaviors they want to include in their routine. The therapist may also want clients to discuss the position they usually sleep in and the combination of pillows and blankets they prefer. Have the clients place the behaviors in the order that seems most convenient and logical to each of them personally. Discuss the routines and how convenient they will be for clients to carry out. Look for any parts of the routine that may get in the way of falling asleep. For example, planning the next day's schedule, assembling clothes to wear, and organizing papers to take to work may take too long and be too mentally arousing to include in a prebedtime routine. Those activities are better placed earlier in the evening. Change the routines as necessary. Record the routines. Make sure the clients have each recorded their personal routine.

Instruct clients to carry out the routines in the same order every night. Tell them to begin getting ready for bed only after they have begun to feel sleepy. Emphasize the importance of monitoring actual presleep behaviors in the future. They will then be able to note progress in establishing a stable prebed routine and to monitor where changes in the routine need to be made.

Assigning Homework

At the end of each session, clients should be reminded of their homework tasks and the importance these assignments play in the overall therapy. The homework for each week is the same: a daily morning sleep diary, a log of the number of times out of bed each night, and a Practice Record containing 6 questions.

SESSION 3

As in Session 2, the first half of this meeting will consist of going over the practice records in detail and troubleshooting any difficulties encountered. The therapist should have the notes made on what specific behaviors each person was going to attempt during the week. Clients should be asked to report specifically on their progress in carrying out their individual assignments. Check to see if they had any problems in establishing a prebedtime routine. Then go on to the following new material for this session.

Discriminating Behaviors Associated with Good and Poor Sleep

> For most people, some activities and events of the day, the evening, and from just before bedtime can affect sleep. Some may have a positive effect, some a negative effect. Most of you are probably already aware of some of the events and behaviors that help or hinder you in sleeping.

Have clients discuss this topic in terms of their own experiences. Generate a list of things that have a negative effect on sleep. Examples might be drinking coffee in the evening, worrying, reading certain kinds of materials, or having discussions on certain topics, such as finances. List things that have a positive effect on sleep, like exercise during the day, an hour of relaxation before bedtime, or pleasant conversation with a spouse late in the evening.

> Sometimes even though you think about possible connections, you miss some that are important. By looking at the data in your Practice Records, you may be able to see connections that you were unaware of, and to discover some things to change in your daily routine.

Present this search through the Practice Records in terms of each client being their own personal scientist or sleuth. Have clients look over their Practice Records to determine their 3 best and 3 worst nights of sleep. Have them examine the records again for only the good nights to highlight any specific patterns. Repeat this process for the poor nights to see if any different patterns exist. You can see that the success of this exercise will be dependent on the accuracy and detail of the Practice Records. Focus primarily on the following 4 areas: (a) activities from dinnertime to bedtime, (b) activities in getting ready for bed, (c) activities carried out in bed, and (d) content of thinking in bed. Conduct a group discussion and help each person find any patterns they may have missed.

Once clients have pinpointed events and behavior associated with a good night of sleep, discuss ways to make these behaviors a part of their daily routine. Be concrete. Get all of the clients to make a committment to change their behavior. Record the changes each client agrees to make. Repeat this process with the behaviors and events associated with a poor night of sleep. Discuss ways to eliminate these events or behaviors. If some interfering event or behavior cannot be eliminated, discuss ways of minimizing its impact. Announce that at the next meeting the group will assess the results of implementing these changes in their routines and then work to fine-tune these changes. End the session by assigning the routine homework. Add to this the importance of working to increase behaviors associated with a good night of sleep and to decrease behaviors associated with a poor night of sleep.

SESSION 4

The first half of this last session will be conducted just like the previous two. Using the Practice Records and the standard format for problem solving, review any difficulties encountered during the week. Specifically address problems with carrying out the sleep hygiene and stimulus control instructions, establishing a prebedtime routine, and discriminating behaviors associated with a good and a poor night of sleep. Then move on to the 2 new topics for this meeting.

Statement of Positive Demand

During this last session, it is time to insert a positive demand to replace the counterdemand. The therapist should reflect that the clients have been engaging in the treatment recommendations for a period of 3 weeks. If they have been faithful and thorough in following through, they have reached the point at which they should begin to see the results of their labors. In the coming weeks, they should find their sleep improving consistently.

Maintenance and Follow-up

Although the fourth week marks the last treatment session, clients should be told that their improvement program is not ending, only the formal teaching part. This last session marks only the beginning of the last week of therapy. They should continue to fill out all the homework forms and diaries during this fourth week and then they can begin to phase out the use of these self-monitoring forms if they wish. However, they should continue to practice all their new routines until they become automatic parts of their behavior. If they find their sleep deteriorating, it is probably because they have lapsed in their dedication to the new behaviors. Prepare the group members to receive a follow-up call and a package of diaries in about 6 weeks. The follow-up serves the purpose of giving the therapist feedback about the continued progress of the group members. Knowing that they will be contacted may also give clients some added motivation to continue their efforts to alleviate their sleep problems. At the time of the follow-up, you can also send a Client Satisfaction form (Table 8.1) asking for reactions to the treatment program, evaluations of current status, and suggestions for future groups. This form was developed by expanding on the format of Larsen, Attkisson, Hargreaves, and Nguyen (1979).

The therapist should also say a few words about how to avoid having an occasional bad night evolve into a pattern of insomnia. Everyone from time to time has one night or a brief period of sleep troubles, especially during periods of increased stress. If they use the techniques that they have learned during those times and especially if they fight against the tendency to develop performance anxiety, they are highly likely to avert any more serious or persistent pattern of sleep disturbance. For those clients who are not showing much improvement at the

Table 8.1. Client Satisfaction

Name_____ Date_____

Please help us to evaluate our program by answering some questions about the treatment for insomnia you received. We are interested in your honest opinions, regardless of whether they may be positive or negative. Please answer all of the questions by circling the appropriate number or writing in the space provided.

1. How *logical* did this treatment seem to you?

1	2	3	4	5
Not logical at all		Somewhat logical		Very logical

2. How would you rate the *quality* of the treatment you received?

1	2	3	4	5
Very poor		Fair		Excellent

3. Did you get the *kind* of treatment you wanted?

1	2	3	4	5
No, definitely not		Somewhat		Yes, definitely

4. If a *friend* had a problem with insomnia, would you recommend this treatment program to her or him?

1	2	3	4	5
No, definitely not		Perhaps		Yes, definitely

5. If, at some time in the *future*, you were to have a serious problem with insomnia, would you be willing to undergo this same treatment again?

1	2	3	4	5
No not willing at all		Perhaps		Yes, very willing

6. How satisfied are you with the *length* of the treatment you received?

1	2	3	4	5
Very dissatisfied		Moderately satisfied		Very satisfied

7. Did you feel that the therapist gave you enough personal *attention*?

1	2	3	4	5
No, not at all		Somewhat		Yes, very much so

8. Did you feel that the therapist was *warm* and *accepting* of your problem?

1	2	3	4	5
No, not at all		Somewhat		Yes, almost always

19. Did the therapist seem *competent* to treat your problem?

1	2	3	4	5
No, not at all competent		Moderately competent		Yes, very competent

10. Do you feel that you still have a problem with *insomnia*?

1	2	3	4	5
Yes, severe problem		Moderate problem		No, no problem at all

11. Did this treatment help you in *other areas* of your life besides insomnia?

    1   2   3   4   5

    No,   Somewhat   Yes, very much

    not at all

If yes, please explain: _____

_____

12. Did this treatment *interfere* with other areas of your life?

    1   2   3   4   5

    No, not   Somewhat   Yes, very much

    at all

If yes, please explain: _____

_____

13. Are you currently taking any prescription or nonprescription *medication* for sleeping problems?   yes   no

If yes, what medication are you taking _____

How many nights per week do you usually take sleeping medication? _____

_____

14. Why do you think this treatment works or does not work? _____

_____

_____

15. Please provide any other comments that will help us to improve our program.

_____

end of treatment, explain that some habits are more difficult to change and more practice may be needed. Four weeks is the average length of time for improvement to become evident; some people take less time and some take more. Review what they have been doing to see if there is complete and consistent utilization of the therapy.

Chapter 9
Miscellaneous Treatment Issues

COMMON TREATMENT PROBLEMS

In our own work we have collected examples of difficult clients and situations that seem to occur with regularity. We have also developed strategies to use when we encounter these difficult treatment problems. One frequent problem is client resistance to following treatment instructions. Fairly obvious manifestations of this resistance are the client who doesn't really try the suggestions but insists that they would not work for him or her, the client who persistently plays devil's advocate with the therapist, and the person who plays the "yes, but . . . " game. Other less obvious resistant behaviors are complaining that the treatment being offered is not what was expected or wanted, claiming to be diligently adhering to treatment though the therapist is doubtful, and wanting to talk at length about tangential issues. The latter can include topics such as dream analysis, folk remedies (like warm milk, calcium, or vitamins), types of mattresses, the usefulness of tryptophan, and magical or easy solutions to sleep problems. Finally, there is a group of clients who will want to spend a lot of time talking about seemingly peripheral personal problems that they claim are related to their loss of sleep. Common examples would be the recent widow who is having trouble making the adjustment to living alone, the person who has serious marital conflicts, and someone who wants to talk about a particularly stressful life and/or job situation.

Our basic response to these kinds of clients is that we are trying to provide a specific treatment for insomnia that has well-established efficacy, unlike many other remedies with which they may be familiar. We are trying to provide this therapy within a limited amount of time to keep the costs low and because most people are busy and have little time to spare. In order to maximize the efficacy of the therapy, we must cover all of the planned material in these 4 brief sessions. Therefore, it is essential that the group not become sidetracked and spend a lot of time on topics that are not a part of this specific intervention.

We want clients to give this treatment their best shot for the full 4 weeks. If by then or shortly thereafter they do not feel they have improved, then they are free to try some other strategy. But as long as they have gone to so much trouble to join this group, it makes sense to work hard and adhere religiously for 4 weeks. Compared to the length of time that most of the group members have suffered from poor sleep, 4 weeks is just a drop in the bucket. What do they have to lose by trying? Even though some aspects of the therapy may cause discomfort or be burdensome, they are designed to reduce the considerable discomfort clients have experienced over a long period of time. We know from a great deal of past experience that adherence to the total treatment package is highly likely to lead to improvement. We also know that nonadherence is almost guaranteed to lead to no change or even to a slight worsening of the sleep problem.

The therapist may be tempted to alter the treatment instructions for those clients who complain or say they cannot comply. The therapist needs to resist strongly any such temptation to reduce expectations for any client. Instead, the therapist should always take a problem-solving stance. The object is to help clients find some way to facilitate compliance with the therapy instructions, not to find ways of reducing demands on the clients. It will be important to discuss the lack of reality in the wish for a magical or effortless cure. Very little that is worth having in life comes without effort. Again we reiterate that long-standing habits cannot be changed without consistent and persistent effort. When you stop to think about it, the fact that many people can reverse the deleterious effects of 20 to 30 years of insomnia with only 4 weeks of hard work is an amazing phenomenon.

Another problem client who is fortunately encountered less often is the person who tries to dominate the proceedings by continuously talking, interrupting, and bullying other members of the group. This person does not really seem interested in making changes in his or her own life. If you encounter such a client, you may have to reduce your efforts toward alleviation of this person's poor sleep. Instead, your efforts may have to be directed at protecting this client from the group's wrath and at minimizing the harm to the rest of the group's progress. The therapist will have to be tactfully assertive and make statements like, "I want others to be sure to have a chance to speak." Try to limit this person's participation in the group. Because this kind of client has no self-control, you will have to provide the control.

The opposite kind of problem is the client who has nothing to say and does not participate in the group. If you cannot get this client to be more active, the group process will be threatened. Push this type of client to participate by asking questions and then relating the material to similarities in what others have already expressed. Another worthwhile tactic is to call on each group member and always be specific. Ask for details even from the person who says that everything is going well.

Finally, from time to time, in spite of your best efforts to screen out disturbed individuals, you will encounter group members who disclose strange and inappropriate or uncomfortable experiences. For example, we have had a client who talked of strange, dreamlike states that she entered, a man who discussed in detail the pornographic audiotapes that he used to relax, and a man who reported having been sexually molested as a child, leaving him afraid of the dark so he now cannot sleep. The therapist needs very quickly to neutralize and redirect these topics before the other group members become alienated. If more subtle attempts within the group session do not eliminate an undesirable behavior, we have found it effective to take a person aside after the session ends. Speak briefly and frankly about how the behavior is interfering with the planned treatment. In most cases, the client is able to control the problem behavior in future sessions. You may want to refer clients for other kinds of help instead of or in addition to behavioral treatment for insomnia.

As an overall tactic, the therapist needs to identify which clients can be counted on for their support of the treatment process. This knowledge will allow the leader to orchestrate the group process. If one person begins to waver and talk of returning to sleeping pills, then the therapist should know what group member to call on who can effectively counter that tendency. If someone insists that the procedures do not work, then call on the client who has been complying and making steady progress. Use group members to help you accomplish the goals of the treatment.

ALTERATIONS FOR THE SLEEP MAINTENANCE CLIENT

Most of the research on behavioral treatment for insomnia focuses on sleep onset problems. Very little attention has been directed toward the nondrug remediation of another kind of sleep disturbance, sleep maintenance insomnia. The latter is usually defined as difficulty returning to sleep after awakening during the night. One reason for this neglect may be the commonly held view that sleep maintenance difficulties are less amenable to treatment than are the more common difficulties of sleep onset insomnia. Behavioral therapy for sleep maintenance problems has been explored in 4 case studies presented by

Thoresen and colleagues (Coates & Thoresen, 1979; Thoresen, Coates, Kirmil-Gray, & Rosekind, 1981), 3 case studies presented by Hoelscher and Edinger (1986), 2 controlled studies by Morin and his colleagues (Morin & Azrin, 1987; Morin et al., 1986), and 3 controlled outcome studies done by our research team (Lacks, Bertelson, Sugerman, & Kunkel, 1983; Davies, Lacks, Storandt, & Bertelson, 1986; Schoicket et al., 1987). From this limited amount of research, it appears that sleep maintenance insomnia is treatable through behavioral methods. In a multiple regression analysis of 216 insomnia sufferers, Lacks and Powlishta (1986) found no differences between amount of treatment success for the sleep onset or the sleep maintenance types.

Furthermore, it appears that stimulus control techniques are also the most effective in relieving sleep maintenance difficulties. This strategy may facilitate the insomniac's return to sleep after arousal because many of the same sleep-interfering behaviors are also taking place during the middle of the night. We had found some support for this idea in our previous work with sleep onset insomniacs. Many of those who had concomitant sleep maintenance problems reported that the stimulus control procedures alleviated both kinds of sleep disturbance (Lacks, Bertelson, Gans, & Kunkel, 1983).

We have used almost the identical stimulus control procedures for the sleep maintenance group as we have with sleep onset insomniacs. The therapist will need to take care to substitute the words "in the middle of the night" for "when you go to bed," "remain asleep" for "fall asleep," and any other phrases that differentiate the two kinds of problems. An example is, "When you wake up during the night, if you find you are unable to fall back asleep, then get up and go into another room." Additional changes in wording will have to be made on some of the evaluation forms. We also emphasize to them that it is normal to wake up several times during the night. It is only a problem if the person becomes too awake and does not fall back asleep quickly. Knowing this helps alleviate performance anxiety associated with awakening in the night. Remember that many poor sleepers suffer from both sleep onset and sleep maintenance difficulties. However, it is our experience that most of these people can easily differentiate which problem is primary or gives them the most discomfort. It is probably best for each treatment group to have members who have the same primary problem.

TREATMENT THROUGH SUCCESSIVE SIEVES

The results of insomnia treatment outcome research for the techniques described in this book have been excellent. However, in spite of this good success, many participants do not attain sleep that falls within the range of that of good sleepers. Insomnia is a complex problem that affects different people in different ways and can be caused by a variety of factors. As such, there are many poor sleepers for whom no single remedy will provide sufficient relief. One possible approach to increased treatment effectiveness is the use of "successive sieves." Using this strategy, each client might first receive the standard stimulus control approach including education in good sleep hygiene, followed by a 1-month practice or consolidation period. After this first stage, those individuals who have not achieved good-sleeper status would be asigned to a second, individualized, symptom-specific condition for 4 weeks, followed by a practice period of the same length. This procedure could then if necessary be repeated a third time.

A program similar to this was used very successfully by Mitchell (1979) to combine muscle relaxation and cognitive control. The combined treatment resulted in 71% SOL reduction in contrast to 40% for muscle relaxation alone. By teaching the skills sequentially with time for consolidation of learning, one might avoid the paradoxical result sometimes found with behavior therapy wherein multiple-component treatments prove less effective than those with a single component. For example Turner, DiTomasso, and Giles (1982) compared sleep onset insomniacs who received either progressive relaxation, stimulus control, or a combination of the two during 4 weeks of therapy. They defined successful treatment outcome as a reduction of SOL to a weekly average of 30 minutes or less. Using this criterion, 60% of the progressive relaxation group, 50% of the stimulus control group, and only 22% of the combined group achieved successful outcome.

The two most appropriate therapies to use as the second and, if necessary, third interventions are cognitive refocusing and progressive relaxation. Which of these two to use — or yet a different method — will depend upon an analysis of the individual needs of each client. Cognitive refocusing has been shown to be equally effective as stimulus control in one study of cognitively aroused insomniacs (T. W. Cook & Lacks, 1986). It may be particularly useful in alleviating sleep disturbance because so many poor sleepers complain of cognitive arousal (Lichstein & Rosenthal, 1980). However, cognitive refocusing is a more difficult procedure to learn for both the therapist and the client. For that reason, it is more desirable to begin with stimulus control techniques that are relatively easy for both therapist and client to master. Also, the skills learned in this approach are ones that most poor sleepers should have in their repertoire. Many of the clients will achieve success sufficient to require no further intervention.

Our model for cognitive refocusing was taken from Turk, Meichenbaum, and Genest (1983) in their work on pain management. The rationale given to clients is that insomnia results from cognitive arousal, that is, the worrying or racing thoughts that insomniacs experience when trying to fall asleep. Bedtime has become associated with cognitive overarousal rather than with relaxation and sleep. Good sleepers are able to put their worries out of their minds and fall asleep quickly. Poor sleepers can get into a vicious cycle of becoming so worried or preoccupied with the possibility of not being able to fall asleep that they actually cause themselves to be more cognitively aroused and thereby make it even more difficult to fall asleep. We frequently use the analogy of test anxiety. The student becomes so worried or anxious about performance on an upcoming test that it is impossible to concentrate and do one's best. Consequently, the student does poorly on the test and is therefore even more worried and anxious before the next exam. This cycle goes on, feeding on itself, until something is done to break it. The therapist is going to help the insomniac break the cycle of cognitive overarousal that leads to one night after another of poor sleep.

The client is told that the core of the treatment will involve learning a number of techniques of visual imagery, distraction, and attention-focusing that can be used to disrupt sleep-incompatible cognitions. These strategies can be engaged in when thoughts interfere with sleep. The concept of competing behaviors is introduced. There are things that individuals cannot do simultaneously, such as using visual imagery and worrying, tossing, and turning in bed. However, to become proficient with these strategies, the client will have to practice them for 30 minutes a day, at any time other than bedtime. During the first week of treatment, the client is asked to practice each of several techniques. By the second week, clients are asked to choose the 1 or 2 strategies that work best for them and to continue to develop their skills in those areas.

Clients are then introduced to imagery techniques and to 3 types of attention focusing. The latter include external focusing, internal focusing, and bodily sensation. For external focus, participants are taught to concentrate attention on such things as their physical surroundings and events outside of themselves, such as a clock ticking or the smell of a scented candle. For internal focus, attention is placed upon a train of thoughts, such as remembering the words to a song or engaging in problems of mental arithmetic (e.g., counting backward from 100 by 7s). In the third type of focus, clients learn to concentrate on the sensations of the body. The concept of attention focusing is what is at work in the old idea of counting sheep. However, counting sheep jumping over a fence is rather boring and so clients will be taught methods that are more attention demanding. Practice sessions in guided imagery aid the client to call forth vivid or pleasant scenarios, such as cutting and then tasting a lemon or a summer beach scene. Additional details of this approach may be found in Turk et al. (1983). Generally, relaxation training alone has not been found to be sufficient to eliminate insomnia. However, it may be a very appropriate adjunct procedure for many poor sleepers. It may help the somatically aroused client or may serve as an additional attention-focusing procedure for the cognitively aroused poor sleeper. Additional details of the procedure for teaching an abbreviated form of muscle relaxation can be found in Bernstein and Borkovec (1973).

SPECIAL ISSUES WITH THE OLDER ADULT

Many practitioners believe that therapeutic procedures developed to treat adults are not applicable to the older adult. Some clinicians hold stereotypical attitudes toward the elderly, seeing them as rigid, unenergetic, and unable to learn new behavior. Their psychological problems are viewed as merely normal representations of old age itself or as the result of irreversible organic disorders. As a result, the elderly are more often treated with medication; nondrug approaches are seen as either unwarranted or impossible (Butler & Lewis, 1982; Dye, 1978; Mintz, Steuer, & Jarvik, 1981).

In contrast to this prevailing attitude, we have not had any negative experience remediating the sleep complaints of the elderly. At first we thought they might respond differently to these techniques than do younger adults. We conducted one early study that was restricted entirely to elderly participants and the results were identical to those from studies in which older adults had been excluded (Puder, Lacks, Bertelson, & Storandt, 1983). Group means on SOL decreased from 68 minutes at baseline to 27 minutes at posttreatment, results that were maintained at a 1-year follow-up. Ten of the 16 insomniacs reduced their sleep latency by 50% or more. Next we thought it would not be wise to mix older and younger adults in the same groups because they might not work well together. Another study thoroughly dispelled that notion (Davies et al., 1986). Since then, we have successfully included individuals up to the age of 78 in a number of studies. We have found that although our older participants begin and end treatment with more sleep disturbance, the degree of response to treatment has been unrelated to the age of the insomnia sufferer. Recently another group of researchers was able to treat successfully older sleep maintenance insomniacs (mean age of 67 years, average duration of 19 years) with behavioral methods. Those who received stimulus control reduced their WASO by 44% after 4 weeks of treatment and by 61% at a 3-month follow-up (Morin et al, 1986).

Because both sleep disturbance and the use of sleep medications increase with age (Miles & Dement, 1980), our results have been very encouraging. Behavior therapy provides a much safer intervention than the more usual practice of prescribing sedative-hypnotic medications. Older people frequently take more than one medication for their multiple chronic health problems. This polypharmacy sets the stage for toxic drug interactions. However, the generalizability of our results is confined to older adults who are independent and self-sufficient as well as relatively well educated. Future researchers will need to explore the effectiveness of behavioral techniques in ameliorating sleep complaints of the institutionalized older person. The majority of older adults, however, are ambulatory. Thus, clinicians can use behavioral strategies for elderly insomniacs, confident that they will respond as well as do younger clients. In addition, the time-limited group approach is suitable, because it is more cost-effective, an important consideration given the financial limitations of many older persons.

In treating geriatric clients, however, one must keep in mind a number of special considerations. Although the elderly are not as different from younger people in as many ways as one may think, certain biological changes do occur with age. Many older adults experience sensory loss, such as impaired vision or hearing, and they may not communicate to the therapist that they have these slight handicaps. The therapist needs to be sensitive to these possible sensory losses and be prepared to make allowances for them. The following suggestions have been made by Davies and Rosenberg (1984) to help minimize the effect of sensory impairment: reduce background noise; speak in the lowest vocal range because low tones are the most audible; be aware of seating arrangements – face-to-face communications are the most easily understood; be sure to have bright overhead lighting and clear copies of handouts. Another important factor is that older clients have a strong fear of traveling when there is bad weather. They are afraid of falling on ice or that cold weather brings a higher risk of illness. Therapists who treat the elderly during wintry weather conditions will need to be much more flexible in scheduling sessions.

These special instructions illustrate the need for those who work with the elderly to take a developmental perspective. Therapists need to be familiar with normal age-related changes and the developmental tasks, crises, and issues of later life. Examples of pertinent issues are bereavement, retirement, dying, and dealing with decreased personal autonomy (Puder, 1984). We have had many women in our insomnia groups who were struggling with the difficult situation of widowhood. Depression with associated sleep problems can be common among the elderly due to loneliness, lack of pleasurable activities, illness and death of friends, and encroaching disability.

Treatments that have shown success with younger clients may have to be modified slightly to achieve the same results with the older client. For example, some older people learn more slowly and their newly learned behaviors may evaporate more rapidly. Treatments may have to be lengthened and proceed more slowly to achieve optimum results (Mintz et al., 1981). The therapist may have to spend more time preparing the client for information, clarifying material, and educating the older client (Puder, 1984). In our own work, we have maintained the standard 4-week program; however, we have sometimes felt that an additional session might have been helpful to our older participants.

Older adults may not be psychologically or scientifically oriented, having received their education in an earlier era. They may not be impressed by the data that support the treatment. Instead, they are more likely to evaluate the worth of the therapy by whether the procedures make sense to them. The therapist should give relatively concrete instructions and use many real-life examples to explain concepts. Furthermore, some groups of older adults prefer the therapist to take the more authoritarian stance of the expert who tells the client what to do.

Bootzin et al. (1983) have also treated many older insomniacs. They report that most of these older adults are highly motivated, an experience that matches our own. These clients are seeking help at a time when their insomnia symptoms are usually severe and have persisted for many years. They enter treatment with a strong intention to comply with the demands of the therapy. However, the treatment protocol that has been described in this book is a complex one that will place many demands on attention and memory. Clients will need a lot of support and reassurance to continue performing all the behaviors required by this therapy over a period of 7 or more weeks. Therapists should consider lack of compliance a problem to be solved rather than a sign of resistance. Clients should be reminded often that the treatment with all its demands is time-limited and worth the most conscientious effort to achieve results. With this type of client, therapists may want to drop some of the evaluation forms that are less essential or to develop abbreviated versions.

We have also found that the attitude and cooperation of the spouse is apparently more important with the elderly insomnia sufferer. Some spouses are not supportive of their partner's attempts to develop new sleep habits. They may not tolerate the poor sleeper who stays out of bed until drowsy or gets out of bed in the middle of the night to read in another room. In just as many cases, however, the client believes the spouse to be unsupportive, but when encouraged to discuss the matter at home, the client finds the spouse to be relatively open to change. With the older client, we have also been faced more often with the question of whether the poor sleeper should move to another bed or another room. It poses a dilemma because we do not want to implement any procedure that might interfere in the client's relationship with the spouse. We will try any number of solutions before agreeing that the client should try sleeping in another room. Even then, we would encourage the client to think of this move as a temporary one; when sleep improves, the client should attempt to move back into the shared bedroom.

Some specific aspects of the behavioral approach to treating insomnia take on added importance with the elderly client. Included among these are education about the "aging of sleep," sleep hygiene, and sleep scheduling. Many older adults are not aware of the natural changes in sleep for their age group, especially the eroding ability to achieve long periods of continuous sleep. Sleep also becomes lighter and more fitful with age. If an older adult is unaware of the changing length and quality of sleep and continues to go to bed at the accustomed hour each night, that person is likely to start waking up at 4 or 5 in the morning. The complaint of insomnia may instead reflect symptoms of frustration, annoyance, and apprehension from spending excessive time in bed trying to get 8 hours of sleep. It is possible that the older person does continue to need about the same amount of sleep as in earlier years but is no longer able to get that amount at any one time due to an inability to sustain sleep in long, unbroken stretches. The problem is one of sleep goals or of sleep efficiency rather than of insufficient sleep. Sleep may just need to be packaged more conveniently (Lichstein & Fischer, 1985). If this is true, stimulus control may be an especially appropriate treatment for the older poor sleeper because it is designed to decrease sleepless time in bed.

Many sleep researchers think that the single most important factor in improving the sleep of the elderly is the regulation of the circadian rhythm. The best way to anchor the sleep-wake schedule is to get up at the same time every morning regardless of the bedtime or amount of sleep the previous night. The elderly frequently stay in bed in the morning because they do not have any pressing reason to get out of bed. They should be encouraged to keep regular schedules of eating, meeting friends, volunteering their time, taking walks, and any other potential activities. Not only will this practice regularize sleep rhythm, it will promote an active, less sedentary, stimulating life that will serve to enhance sleep.

On the other hand, our usual practice of prohibiting napping may not be as appropriate when treating older poor sleepers. A regular afternoon nap may aid these people in gaining more sleep without interfering with their nighttime rest. Naps may be especially desirable for the older person who cannot sustain a high energy level all day. However, afternoon naps are likely to decrease the length of nighttime sleep. Naps would therefore be less appropriate for those who are distressed by short sleep at night or by being awake while others sleep. In any case, naps should not total more than 1 hour per day and should be taken at about the same time each day.

Other good sleep hygiene practices may be more crucial to the older poor sleeper. Sensitivity to caffeine increases with age. Noise may interfere with sleep more in older age; a sound-masking machine may reduce the problem. The body's temperature-regulating mechanisms are less efficient so that feeling cold in bed can interfere with sleep. Gastric reflux problems may require avoiding food in the evening and propping up the mattress to keep the head elevated during sleep. Diuretics taken for hypertension can cause frequent awakenings to urinate, this situation may be helped by cutting down on fluids in the evening. Certain medications for medical disorders can delay sleep onset if taken in the evening. Many older adults do not feel secure in their homes at night and so cannot sleep. Special attention to burglar and fire security is one way to alleviate this anxiety (American Medical Association, 1984).

CHILD AND ADOLESCENT SLEEPING DISORDERS

Much less is known about the sleep disorders of children and adolescents. Anyone who works with adult insomniacs, however, is aware that a certain percentage of them report having first developed their sleep problems as a child or even at birth. A study of 629 high school seniors revealed that about 13% of adolescents report suffering from chronic insomnia and an additional 38% complain of occasional poor sleep (Price et al., 1978). Coates and Thoresen (1981) describe other survey findings documenting child and adolescent sleep problems. In one study, pediatricians and child psychiatrists reported on the incidence of sleep complaints in their practice. Pediatricians found that 26% of their practice had sleep complaints; child psychiatrists found 61%. Of these 5% and 19%, respectively, had insomnia, 8% and 11% enuresis, 8% and 18% nightmares, and 2% and 6% night terrors. Only small percentages complained of hypersomnia, narcolepsy, and somnambulism. Another study suggests that many people may begin to use sleep medication in adolescence. In a random sample of 12-to-17-year-olds, 3% reported using a sedative or tranquilizer during the past month and 7% used such medication during the past year. In a group of high school seniors who reported chronic sleeplessness, 20% had begun at least the occasional use of sleep medications.

One comparison of childhood onset with adult onset insomnia found that the former took longer to fall asleep and slept for shorter periods of time than the latter who showed more restless sleep (Hauri & Olmstead, 1980). Those who developed their sleep disorder during adulthood could usually name a specific psychological stress that occurred around the onset of their sleep difficulties, whereas most of the childhood onset group could not. Although most of those with childhood onset insomnia felt that their sleep problems were relatively constant, the adult-onset group felt that their sleep problems fluctuated with their mood or level of stress. Based upon sleep patterns in the laboratory and upon interviews, Hauri and Olmstead found more soft neurological signs in the childhood onset group. They speculated that these insomniacs may have some neurological impairment in the structures that relate to the sleep-wake balance. Adult onset insomniacs are more likely to have had psychological or conditioning factors lead to their sleep disturbance. If these findings are borne out by further research, childhood onset insomnia may prove to be less amenable to treatment with current methods.

For adolescents the negative effects of sleep disturbance are similar to those of adults: irritability, depression, poor self-image, and problems with school attendance and performance. In spite of these deleterious effects, children are unlikely to receive treatment for their sleep disorders, and researchers have given the topic scant attention. The few studies that have treated young children have focused primarily on parent behavior. Child sleep disturbance can frequently be traced to high levels of maternal anxiety, inconsistent handling, and overresponsiveness to child night waking. These parents often respond to child waking by feeding, handling, or bringing the child into the parental bed. Parental anger about child waking seems to compound the sleeping disturbance (Coates & Thoresen, 1981).

Largo and Hunziker (1984) conducted a 2- to 6-week treatment program for the parents of 52 sleep disturbed children ages 24 to 36 months. Parents monitored their child's sleep on a daily sleep chart, received education and counseling about their child's sleep, and learned to set realistic expectations. Over one third of the parents were able to resolve the sleep problems solely through sleep monitoring. Another 47% did so with the combination of monitoring and counseling. Other treatment studies of young children have used behavioral techniques such as withdrawal of parental attention to a wakeful child, positive reinforcement for the desired behavior, development of a bedtime ritual, and shaping the child's behavior. With older children, treatment has more often focused on the sleep-disturbed child's use of techniques like relaxation training (e.g., Kirmil-Gray, Coates, Thoresen, & Rosekind, 1978; Weil & Goldfried, 1973).

Perhaps one of the most promising approaches is found in a recent book on helping the child sleep through the night that is directed to the parents of children from infancy to age 5 (Cuthbertson & Schevill, 1985). The book presents a parent training program for the development from birth of a healthy infant sleeping pattern. Parents are taught through concrete suggestions to help their infant to form early, consistent, and lasting good sleeping habits. Parents learn to use a step-by-step behavioral strategy that takes into account the child's nutritional and emotional needs but at the same time avoids methods that will interfere with the child's development of healthy and self-sufficient sleep patterns.

In our own work (Wolfson, 1987), we are currently investigating the utility of this approach with 60 sets of first-time parents; half are receiving the behavioral program and half are only monitoring their newborn's sleep. Participants attend 4 60-to-90-minute sessions, 2 prenatal and 2 postnatal. In the first 2 meetings parents receive didactic information on infant and child sleep, such as sleep-waking patterns, the association between feeding and sleeping, basic physiology of sleep, confident parenting, and the importance of establishing an early sleep routine for the infant. Parents also learn a set of behaviors to get their child on the right track before the infant is developmentally ready to sleep through the night. Parents are instructed not to hold or feed their infant to sleep, to gradually concentrate wake time in day hours, to develop a focal feeding time between 10 p.m. and midnight, and not to rush to pick up an infant who signals at night, but to see if the baby can return to sleep independently.

When the child is developmentally ready to sleep through the night (at about age 5 to 6 weeks), parents receive 2 booster sessions to review material and problem solve. At this time they initiate a 4-night, step-by-step approach to lengthen gradually the baby's nighttime sleeping period. Follow-up measures of the baby's sleep and the parents' level of stress and parental self-efficacy are being collected when the babies are 4 months of age. It may be that if parents can learn to help their child develop independence at night, pediatricians and child psychiatrists will see fewer cases of children with sleep disturbance.

Chapter 10
Current Assessment and Future Directions

From the material presented earlier in this book, it is clear that insomnia is not a unitary concept, but is instead very complex. Although we know a great deal about sleep disorders, there is even more that we do not know. The complaint of insomnia is a symptom, not a disorder. This complaint can take many forms, such as trouble falling asleep, remaining asleep, or waking too early in the morning. The complaint can also originate from numerous different psychological as well as physical causes. The Association of Sleep Disorders Centers diagnostic system lists 65 different diagnostic categories of sleep disturbance, only 9 of which are considered to be forms of insomnia. No one treatment is appropriate for all of these categories of sleep disturbance. Some types will need a strictly medical approach, some will benefit by psychological intervention, and others may best be helped by a combination of approaches. An accurate differential diagnosis is essential for intelligent treatment planning. The two diagnostic categories of sleep-onset insomnia of the psychophysiological and subjective subtypes appear to be the most appropriate for the application of behavioral approaches.

A number of different behavioral approaches have grown out of a handful of theoretical interpretations of the cause of these two subtypes of insomnia. Those who advocate a somatic hyperarousal theory endorse the use of various relaxation methods such as progressive relaxation and biofeedback. Emphasis on the effects of performance anxiety on sleep leads to the use of paradoxical intention. Those who believe that operant conditioning serves to create and maintain insomnia turn to stimulus control techniques. An emphasis on the cognitive hyperarousal theory leads logically to the use of cognitive refocusing or guided imagery. At this point in the study of insomnia, we cannot say which of these competing theories is the most accurate or even which applies to an individual case of poor sleep. All have face validity and some offer empirical support.

Although the clinical utility of these techniques has been established, there is no clear understanding of the elusive mechanism of change for the various methods. Often the theoretical underlying process does not appear to be operating during empirical trials. For example, Woolfolk and McNulty (1983) found little evidence to support the view that improvements gained from progressive relaxation are due to reduced muscle tension. Instead of decreases in autonomic hyperactivity, reductions of cognitive intrusions have been observed to parallel improved sleep obtained with progressive relaxation (e.g., Mitchell, 1979). It may be that in the process of training for relaxation, participants learn to focus their attention on relatively pleasant, monotonous, internal sensations that are incompatible with the cognitive arousal that interferes with sleep (Borkovec, 1982).

As for stimulus control, good and poor sleepers have not usually been found to differ on amount of sleep-incompatible behaviors in the bed or bedroom (e.g., Haynes et al., 1982). In addition, Zwart and Lisman (1979) found that they could produce equal therapeutic outcome with stimulus control or with countercontrol techniques, the latter of which required the sleepless subject to remain in the bed and to engage in sleep-incompatible behaviors. They concluded that both treatments "contingently disrupt sleep-incompatible activities and/or cognitions that occur during the difficult period prior to sleep onset" (p. 117). Both stimulus control and countercontrol treatment procedures have in common the disruption of a pattern of behaviors that have been associated with nonsleep. That is, the person no longer lies in bed trying to fall asleep and meeting with no success (i.e., no reward). Instead, the person engages in behaviors that are unrelated to sleep (reading, watching television). It may be that other methods are also effective in disrupting the association of the bed with nonsleep.

Borkovec (1982) has attempted to show how all of these theories can be combined to explain the typical case of insomnia. The poor sleeper experiences intrusive, relatively uncontrollable cognitive arousal that is similar to what we might call worry and that may lead to CNS arousal. These presleep and during-sleep cognitions lead to a distorted perception of the passage of time and a subjective experience of wakefulness during early stages of sleep and during the lighter stages of sleep later on in the night. One source of this cognitive arousal is the tense, obsessive style often found among poor sleepers. Interpersonal conflicts and environmental stress exacerbate the person's tendency toward cognitive arousal. However, these factors ebb and flow during the week and may be the source of the high variability of sleep experienced by the insomnia sufferer. Other worrisome cognitions may develop as the person begins to fret over the loss of sleep. As more and more frustrating time is spent in the bed attempting to fall asleep, the bed and bedroom may become aversively associated with cognitive arousal and with other sleep-incompatible behaviors that further maintain the sleep problems.

It may be that each of the most frequently used treatments for insomnia has some measure of success because each addresses to some degree a causative factor that can be found in many or most poor sleepers. Or they may all work because they share some common process, such as the reduction or prevention of arousing, sleep-preventing cognitions or the direction of attention away from these cognitions. The latter speculation is lent support because improvement in sleep has been shown to be associated with the reduction of cognitive intrusions — even when the therapy used is progressive relaxation or stimulus control.

Another issue is the amount of improvement clients experience from the application of these behavioral strategies. Although many studies report group averages of reduced sleeplessness, not all individuals are helped equally by these treatments. One person may drop from 200 minutes SOL to 100 minutes, still showing a considerable disturbance of sleep. Another may drop from 60 minutes to 30 minutes, a figure that approaches the range of good sleepers. Some may show minimal or no change, whereas others greatly exceed the overall group improvement rate. Group means only obscure this variability. Reductions of target behaviors that are reported to be of *statistical* significance may also be so small as to be of minimal *clinical* merit. Unfortunately, outcome data are rarely reported in a format that allows others, especially practitioners, to judge the likelihood that a procedure will substantially eliminate an individual's problem behavior. When insomnia researchers have provided information on clinical outcomes, they have not done so in a consistent or rigorous manner.

Recently N. S. Jacobson, Follette, and Revenstorf (1984) challenged clinical researchers to provide "information about the effects of psychotherapy which is both clinically meaningful and statistically reliable" (p.337). For maximum utility, they urge researchers to use agreed-upon conventions that are psychometrically sound and applicable to a wide variety of clinical problems. They propose that improvement in therapy is clinically significant when the client makes a change that is both statistically reliable (i.e., exceeds chance expectations) and that returns the client to normative levels of functioning on whatever variable is being used to measure the clinical problem.

To assess clinical significance of our own work, we reanalyzed using a standardized protocol the data from 7 outcome studies of behavior therapy for insomnia done over a 4-year period by our research team. Generally, each study varied only in the use of individuals whose primary complaint was either sleep onset or sleep maintenance insomnia and in the content of treatments used. From these 7 outcome studies, we assembled a pool of 216 former participants, 129 of whom had been treated for a primary complaint of sleep onset insomnia and 87 for sleep maintenance problems (Lacks & Powlishta, 1986). We had available a short-term follow-up (6 to 12 weeks) for all the participants and a 1-year long-term follow-up for about half of them. As had been shown previously in each of the 7 individual studies of this reanalysis, insomnia sufferers as a group were able to achieve and to maintain highly statistically significant reductions in their sleep complaint. These group figures, however, do not reflect the progress of the individual insomnia sufferers.

To look at response to treatment on an individual basis, the data for each participant were examined for the intervals between baseline and each of the 3 other times of measurement (end of treatment, short-term follow-up and year follow-up) and during the interval between end of treatment and short-term follow-up. Each subject was classified as improved, unchanged, or deteriorated during each of these 4 intervals by using an index of statistically reliable change. To meet this criterion of statistically significant change, an increase or decrease of 37 minutes SOL or 49 minutes WASO was needed.

The second prong of the analysis of individual outcomes was to determine clinically meaningful progress. To be judged to have evidenced clinically significant improvement, individuals were required both to show change that exceeded chance expectations and to move into the range of good sleepers. The nondistressed range for both SOL and WASO was operationalized as falling within 2 standard deviations above the mean SOL or WASO of good sleepers. These good sleeper means and standard deviations were obtained by pooling data from 5 studies that reported SOL ($n = 65$, M - 11.99 minutes, $SD = 6.5$) and 3 studies that reported WASO ($n = 27$, $M = 8.7$ minutes, $SD = 11.01$). Cutoff values were 25 and 31 minutes for SOL and WASO, respectively. In other words, persons who reduced their average SOL to 25 minutes or less or average WASO to 31 minutes or less, were judged to have attained good sleeper status. This dual criterion for clinically significant improvement was used to prevent the spurious inflation of the results by individuals who were close to the good sleeper range before treatment began.

After 4 weeks of behavior therapy for insomnia, 43% of all the participants demonstrated real improvement in their sleep complaint. By the short-term follow-up, another 15% began to or continued to improve beyond their posttest levels. From baseline to short-term follow-up, 51% of the insomniacs had improved reliably. Deterioration rates were low: less than 1% at posttest, about 3% from posttest to short-term follow-up, and none from baseline to the 1-year follow-up. The rest of the subjects showed no reliable change in their sleep complaint. As for clinically significant change, overall 29% of participants showed resolution of their presenting problem after 4 weeks of treatment; by short-term follow-up 32% had achieved this status. Complaints of delayed sleep latency and trouble maintaining sleep remitted at about equal rates. However, clients who received stimulus control had an initial treatment advantage over those who received some other behavior therapy (49% vs. 39% improved at posttreatment). This advantage disappeared sometime during the 4 to 12 weeks following treatment. In addition, individuals who were younger, as well as those who experienced their first episode of insomnia at a later age, those who had insomnia for a longer time, and those who evidenced less psychopathology were each found to have an initial treatment advantage that disappeared sometime during the 4 to 12 weeks following therapy.

Using these stringent evalutive criteria, our success rates have been rather modest. Of the insomniacs we treated, a substantial proportion of those who demonstrated real change continued to have levels of sleep disturbance that would be classified as insomnia. On the other hand, deterioration rates were low, and good maintenance of improvement was found for periods of up to a year. How do these conservative criteria of treatment success compare with other standards? At the 1-year follow-up we had information on 5 different critera for improvement: (a) statistically reliable improvement (48%), (b) clinically significant improvement or real change combined with becoming a good sleeper (30%), (c) at least a 50% reduction of initial sleep complaint (52%), (d) clients who label themselves as no longer having insomnia (36%), and (e) absence of sleep medication (76%). The last point is important information because behavioral treatment specifically aims to eliminate the need for hypnotic medication. At baseline, 35% of our volunteers were using sleep medication on an average of 3 nights a week and had been doing so for an average of 7 years. Success rates using these standards differed considerably, ranging from 30% for eradication of the sleep problem to 76% for a sleep-medication-free state.

From these various criteria, it appears that, following behavior therapy, about 50% of insomnia sufferers do show some kind of real change using a variety of criteria. Researchers in this area need not be discouraged by these results. Even if only a small proportion of the insomniacs in our research attained good sleeper status, a minimal expenditure of professional time allowed many to reduce the degree and extent of their sleep complaint (on the average by over 35 minutes per night and from 5 to 2 nights per week). Overall, clients seemed very pleased with their progress and reported greatly enhanced self-efficacy. Once attained, their better sleep skills were stable. These results should be viewed in the context that chronic insomniacs who do not receive treatment do not experience spontaneous remission. The average duration of sleep disturbance among our subjects was 13 years and ranged upward to 40 years. Researchers in other areas, such as behavioral marital therapy (e.g. N. S. Jacobson et al., 1984b) or headache relief (e.g., Blanchard & Andrasik, 1985) have reported greater levels of initial response but much lower maintenance of therapy gains.

However, those of us who are concerned about this particular clinical problem must not be entirely satisfied with these results. Strategies will need to be developed to make currently available interventions more therapeutic to larger numbers of poor sleepers and to devise new treatment methods. Perhaps longer therapy into which new information and techniques are introduced would be helpful. However, the addition of booster sessions with more practice but no new information does not seem to enhance outcome (M. A. Cook & Lacks, 1984). Many researchers in this area have noted large individual differences in susceptibility to the available methods. They have called for attempts to match individually tailored techniques with specific client characteristics. However, little is known about the mechanisms of change and their relationship to client variables, making it difficult to individualize treatment.

Hauri (1981) treated poor sleepers who were randomly assigned to either EMG or SMR biofeedback. Disappointed with the results, he went back and classified each subject as having received either an "appropriate" or "inappropriate" treatment on the basis of information collected at baseline. EMG training was assumed to be appropriate for tense, anxious individuals, and SMR training was considered best for those having poor sleep patterns and disrupted sleep. When the results were reanalyzed, only those participants who received an appropriate treatment improved their sleep problem; inappropriate biofeedback did not reduce sleep complaint.

Our own initial attempt to use a symptom-specific intervention did not increase success rates. Cognitively aroused insomniacs who received cognitive refocusing did not benefit any more than those who were treated with stimulus control (T. W. Cook & Lacks, 1986). However,

this strategy appears to be one still worth pursuing. Many of our participants continue to complain after therapy that they are plagued by
nighttime cognitive intrusions. Several researchers have reported that
increased nighttime cognitive arousal in insomniacs may be associated
with higher than normal daytime physical hypoactivity due to a more
sedentary lifestyle (de la Peña, 1978: Marchini et al., 1983). Strategies to
alter daytime behaviors rather than focusing on nighttime activities
could be a promising new avenue in the treatment of insomnia.

There exist several limits to the generalization from the research
findings of the behavioral treatment of insomnia. Participants in these
studies tend to be female, white, middle-class, and well educated.
These clients are likely to be ones who want a nondrug treatment that
emphasizes self-responsibility and self-control. A less educated, clinic
population may produce different results. Surveys also indicate that
insomnia is more prevalent among individuals of low educational and
socioeconomic status (e.g., Bixler et al., 1979). Our own clients have also
been all adults, making questionable any generalization of our results to
treatment for children and adolescents. Given the finding that those
who develop insomnia at an early age may be less amenable to
treatment, more attention to childhood insomnia is in order. Another
issue is that our treatments were always given in small groups. Based
on a handful of cases we have treated individually, the accountability
and support offered by the group appear to be powerful therapeutic
elements. Because treatment in clinical settings is more likely to be
administered to individuals than to groups, the differential effectiveness of these two modes of providing therapy should be examined.

Our clients, as well as those in most other outcome studies, were also
well screened to eliminate depression, other psychopathology, physical
illness, and chronic pain — all conditions that are often associated with
sleeping difficulties. Little is known about how behavior therapy for
insomnia would work within these other contexts. Depression is
probably the most obvious example of a disorder in which sleep
disturbance plays a prominent part. The conventional attitude is that
when the depression is treated and is relieved, the sleep complaints will
show concomitant improvements. However, we know that insomnia
can often develop a functional autonomy from its original source and be
maintained by factors such as conditioning or performance anxiety. To
prevent the development of persistent insomnia, it may be wise to offer
a separate adjunct treatment for sleep disturbance that is thought to be
secondary to psychopathology. Although it was not strictly an intervention for insomnia, one group of researchers found that when they
restricted the caffeine intake of psychiatric inpatients they found
clinically significant reductions in enuresis, insomnia, and behaviors
requiring restraint (Edelstein et al., 1984).

Medical patients with secondary insomnia are routinely given pharmacological treatment. For example, 44% of all psychotropic drug prescriptions in 5 major oncology treatment centers were for disturbed sleep (Derogatis et al., 1979). Stam and Bultz (1986) report that the fatigue, irritability, and depressed mood that often accompany insomnia can greatly affect the quality of life of cancer patients. They treated a 27-year-old man with severe insomnia secondary to cancer and chemotherapy. A combination of somatic focusing and imagery training was presented in 5 weekly sessions. SOL fell from 1.9 hours at baseline to .7 hours at week 4, and to .3 hours at a 1-year follow-up. Duration of sleep went from about 4 to 7 hours per night.

In another study (Cannici, Malcolm, & Peek, 1983), 15 adult cancer inpatients and outpatients were given muscle relaxation training in individual sessions on 3 consecutive days; another 15 patients received routine medical care. The group that was given behavior therapy reduced SOL from 124 to 29 minutes, and the control group had SOL means that went from 116 to 104 minutes. Experimental patients increased their hours of sleep by about 90 minutes per night. These results were observed during the 3 days after the 3-day intervention and were almost identical to those obtained at a follow-up 3 months later. Six of the treated patients reduced their SOL to less than 15 minutes and 90% showed noticeable improvement. Outpatients appeared to profit more than inpatients. The researchers speculated that the muscle-relaxation technique provided a distraction from the pain or may have loosened tightened muscle groups that were producing or increasing pain. Other less obvious medical groups that show sleep disturbance include those with asthma, kidney disease, kidney transplants, severe eczema, and hyperthyroidism (R. L. Williams, 1978). An important future direction for insomnia researchers and practitioners will be to see if our behavioral approaches can serve as adjunct therapies for sleep disturbance secondary to medical conditions.

Finally, the results of these studies are based on the subjective aspects of insomnia that have not been validated against EEG-defined sleep. Although improvements in self-report following progressive relaxation have been verified a number of times by polysomnography (Borkovec, 1982), no such research has been done for other strategies like stimulus control or cognitive refocusing. However, Morin et al. (1986) found that reductions in awakening duration and sleep latency, following both stimulus control and imagery training, were corroborated by an electromechanical timer. Because it is the complaint of insomnia that leads an individual to seek remediation, this behavior appears to be a central feature of insomnia and thus an appropriate target for treatment. However, future sleep laboratory investigations of these issues are indicated in order to generalize results to objectively defined sleep.

In summary, future directions for research and practice should aim toward (a) a greater understanding of the conditions that cause insomnia, (b) understanding the mechanisms for change that underlie behavior therapy, (c) attempts to tailor therapy to the individual poor sleeper, (d) application of behavioral techniques to a broader group of clients, (e) attention to remediation of the sleep problems of children and adolescents, and (f) trials of behavioral methods as adjunct treatments for insomnia secondary to psychiatric and medical conditions.

Recommended Readings

American Medical Association. (1984). *Guide to better sleep*. New York: Random House.

Association of Sleep Disorders Centers. (1979). Diagnostic classification of sleep and arousal disorders. *Sleep, 2*, 1–137.

Bootzin, R. R., & Nicassio, P. M. (1978). Behavioral treatments for insomnia. In M. Hersen, R. Eisler, & P. Miller (Eds.), *Progress in behavior modification* (Vol. 6, pp. 1–45). New York: Academic Press.

Bootzin, R. R., Engle-Friedman, M., & Hazelwood, L. (1983). Insomnia. In P. M. Lewinsohn, & L. Teri (Eds.), *Clinical geropsychology: New directions in assessment and treatment* (pp. 81–115). New York: Pergamon.

Borkovec, T. D. (1982). Insomnia. *Journal of Consulting and Clinical Psychology, 50*, 880–895.

Dement, W. C. (1976). *Some must watch while some must sleep*. San Francisco: Freeman.

Appendices

APPENDIX A. SCORING INSTRUCTIONS FOR THE SLEEP HYGIENE AWARENESS AND PRACTICE SCALE (SHAPS)

Sleep Hygiene Knowledge
Correct answer = 1 point   Item omitted = 2 points   Incorrect answer = 3 points

Items 1–6, 9, and 13 are disruptive of sleep.
If responses to these questions are: 1, 2, 3, or 4, score as incorrect.
                                        5, 6, or 7, score as correct.

Items 7, 8, 10, 11, and 12 are beneficial to sleep.
If responses to these questions are: 1, 2, or 3, score as correct.
                                        4, 5, 6, or 7, score as incorrect.

Note: the response 4 is always incorrect.
Scores on this section may range from 13–39. Higher scores indicate less sleep hygiene knowledge.

Caffeine Knowledge
The following are the correct answers:

N 7-Up soft drink	N lemonade	Y Mountain Dew
Y regular tea	N root beer	Y cola soft drinks
Y Dristan cold remedy	Y chocolate cake	Y Dexatrim diet pills
N aspirin	Y regular coffee	N Tylenol
Y Dr. Pepper soft drink	Y Excedrin	Y Aqua Ban diuretic
Y Midol menstrual relief	Y Sudafed decongestant	N Sprite soft drink

The score is the number correct divided by the number answered and then multiplied by 100.

Scores may range from 0 to 100. A higher score indicates better knowledge of caffeine.

Sleep Hygiene Practice
The total score is the sum of the answers to all the items; reverse the scores for items 16–19 (i.e., 0 = 7, 1 = 6, 2 = 5, 3 = 4, 4 = 3, 5 = 2, 6 = 1, 7 = 0).

Scores may range from 0 to 133; higher scores indicate less healthy sleep hygiene practice.

APPENDIX B. PRACTICE RECORD — STIMULUS CONTROL

Name _____
Week Number _____

How sleepy were you when you first went to bed last night?	What time did you get up this morning?	Briefly list your activities in getting ready for bed.	Briefly list your activities from dinner to bedtime.	List any activities you carried out in bed yesterday.	What were you thinking about in bed last night?
MONDAY 1 2 3 4 5 Not Sleepy Very Sleepy					
TUESDAY 1 2 3 4 5 Not Sleepy Very Sleepy					
WEDNESDAY 1 2 3 4 5 Not Sleepy Very Sleepy					

143

THURSDAY

1   2   3   4   5

Not   Very
Sleepy   Sleepy

FRIDAY

1   2   3   4   5

Not   Very
Sleepy   Sleepy

SATURDAY

1   2   3   4   5

Not   Very
Sleepy   Sleepy

SUNDAY

1   2   3   4   5

Not   Very
Sleepy   Sleepy

APPENDIX C. TIMES OUT OF BED
HOMEWORK SHEET

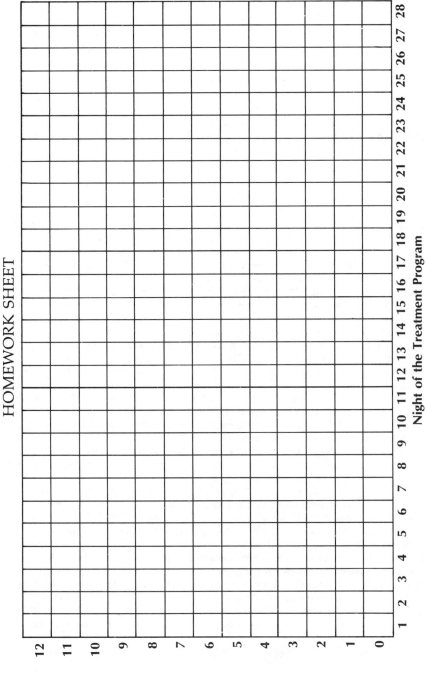

Night of the Treatment Program

Number of Times Out of Bed

References

American Medical Association. (1984). *Guide to better sleep*. New York: Random House.

American Psychiatric Association. (1980). *Diagnostic and statistical manual of mental disorders* (3rd ed.). Washington, DC: Author.

Ascher, L. M. (1980). Paradoxical intention. In A. Goldstein & E. B. Foa (Eds.), *Handbook of behavioral interventions: A clinical guide* (pp. 266–321). New York: Wiley.

Aserinsky, E., & Kleitman, N. (1953). Regularly occurring periods of eye motility and concomitant phenomena during sleep. *Science, 118*, 273–274.

Association of Sleep Disorders Centers. (1979). Diagnostic classification of sleep and arousal disorders. *Sleep, 2*, 1–137.

Baekeland, F., & Lasky, R. (1966). Exercise and sleep patterns in college athletes. *Perceptual and Motor Skills, 23*, 1203–1207.

Beck, A. T. (1967). *Depression: Clinical, experimental, and theoretical aspects*. New York: Harper & Row.

Bernstein, D. A., & Borkovec, T. D. (1973). *Progressive relaxation training: A manual for the helping professions*. Champaign, IL: Research Press.

Bertelson, A. D. (1984). *Drugs commonly prescribed as hypnotics or tranquilizers*. Unpublished document, Washington University, St. Louis, MO.

Beutler, L. E., Thornby, J. I., & Karacan, I. (1978). Psychological variables in the diagnosis of insomnia. In R. L. Williams & I. Karacan (Eds.), *Sleep disorders: Diagnosis and treatment* (pp. 61–100). New York: Wiley.

Bixler, E. O., Kales, J. D., Scharf, M. B., Kales, A., & Leo, L. A. (1976). Incidence of sleep disorders in medical practice: A physician survey. *Sleep Research, 5*, 62.

Bixler, E. O., Kales, A., Soldatos, C. R., Kales, J. D., & Healey, E. S. (1979). Prevalence of sleep disorders in the Los Angeles metropolitan area. *American Journal of Psychiatry, 136*, 1257–1262.

Blanchard, E. B., & Andrasik, F. (1985). *Management of chronic headaches: A psychological approach*. New York: Pergamon.

Bootzin, R. R. (1972). Stimulus control treatment for insomnia [Summary]. *Proceedings of the 80th Annual Convention of the American Psychological Association, 7*, 395–396.

Bootzin, R. R. (1977). Effects of self-control procedures for insomnia. In R. Stuart (Ed.), *Behavioral self-management: Strategies, techniques, and outcome* (pp. 176–195). New York: Brunner/Mazel.

Bootzin, R. R., & Engle-Friedman, M. (1981). The assessment of insomnia. *Behavioral Assessment, 3*, 107–126.

Bootzin, R. R., Engle-Friedman, M., & Hazelwood, L. (1983). Insomnia. In P. M. Lewinsohn & L. Teri (Eds.), *Clinical geropsychology: New directions in assessment and treatment* (pp. 81–115). New York: Pergamon.

146

Bootzin, R. R., & Nicassio, P. M. (1978). Behavioral treatments for insomnia. In M. Hersen, R. Eisler, & P. Miller (Eds.), *Progress in behavior modification* (Vol. 6, pp. 1–45). New York: Academic Press.

Borkovec, T. D. (1982). Insomnia. *Journal of Consulting and Clinical Psychology, 50,* 880–895.

Borkovec, T. D., Lane, T. W., & VanOot, P. H. (1981). Phenomenology of sleep among insomniacs and good sleepers: Wakefulness experience when cortically asleep. *Journal of Abnormal Psychology, 90,* 607–609.

Borkovec, T. D., & Nau, S. D. (1972). Credibility of analogue therapy rationales. *Journal of Behavior Therapy and Experimental Psychiatry, 3,* 257–260.

Borkovec, T. D., & Weerts, T. C. (1976). Effects of progressive relaxation on sleep disturbance: An electroencephalographic evaluation. *Psychosomatic Medicine, 38,* 173–180.

Butler, R., & Lewis, M. (1982). *Aging and mental health.* St. Louis, MO: Mosby.

Cannici, J., Malcolm, R., & Peek, L. A. (1983). Treatment of insomnia in cancer patients using muscle relaxation training. *Journal of Behavior Therapy and Experimental Psychiatry, 14,* 251–256.

Carrington, P. (1977). *Freedom in meditation.* New York: Anchor/Doubleday.

Carskadon, M. A., Dement, W. C., Mitler, M. M., Guilleminault, C., Zarcone, V. P., & Spiegel, R. (1976). Self-reports vs. sleep laboratory findings in 122 drug-free subjects with complaints of chronic insomnia. *American Journal of Psychiatry, 133,* 1382–1388.

Coates, T. J., Killen, J. D., George, J., Silverman, S., Marchini, E., & Thoresen, C. E. (1982). Estimating sleep parameters: A multitrait-multimethod analysis. *Journal of Consulting and Clinical Psychology, 50,* 345–352.

Coates, T. J., & Thoresen, C. E. (1977). *How to sleep better: A drug-free program for overcoming insomnia.* Englewood Cliffs, NJ: Prentice-Hall.

Coates, T. J., & Thoresen, C. E. (1979). Treating arousals during sleep using behavioral self-management. *Journal of Consulting and Clinical Psychology, 47,* 603–605.

Coates, T. J., & Thoresen, C. E. (1981). Sleep disturbance in children and adolescents. In E. G. Mash & L. G. Terdal (Eds.), *Behavioral assessment of childhood disorders* (pp. 639–678). New York: Guilford.

Coleman, R. M. et al. (1982). Sleep-wake disorders based on a polysomnographic diagnosis. *Journal of the American Medical Association, 247,* 997–1003.

Cook, M. A., & Lacks, P. (1984, November). The effectiveness of booster sessions in the treatment of sleep onset insomnia. Paper presented at the annual meeting of the Association for the Advancement of Behavior Therapy, Philadelphia, PA.

Cook, T. W., & Lacks, P. (1986). *Insomnia and cognitive arousal: The effectiveness of a symptom-specific treatment.* Manuscript submitted for publication.

Coursey, R. D., Buchsbaum, M., & Frankel, B. L. (1975). Personality measures and evoked responses in chronic insomniacs. *Journal of Abnormal Psychology, 84,* 239–249.

Cox, D. J., Freundlich, A., & Meyer, R. G. (1975). Differential effectiveness of electromyographic feedback, verbal relaxation instructions, and medication placebo with tension headaches. *Journal of Consulting and Clinical Psychology, 43,* 892–898.

Cuthbertson, J., & Schevill, S. (1985). *Helping your child sleep through the night.* New York: Doubleday.

Davies, R., Lacks, P., Storandt, M., & Bertelson, A. D. (1986). Countercontrol treatment of sleep maintenance insomnia in relation to age. *Psychology and Aging, 1,* 233–238.

Davies, R., & Rosenberg, A. (1984). *Guidelines for behavior therapy with older adult poor sleepers.* Unpublished manuscript, Washington University, St. Louis, MO.

Davison, G. C., Tsujimoto, R. N., & Glaros, A. G. (1973). Attribution and the maintenance of behavior change in falling asleep. *Journal of Abnormal Psychology, 82,* 124–133.

de la Peña, A. (1978). Toward a psychophysiologic conceptualization of insomnia. In R. L. Williams & I. Karacan (Eds.), *Sleep disorders: Diagnosis and treatment* (pp. 101–143). New York: Wiley.

Dement, W. C. (1976). *Some must watch while some must sleep.* San Francisco: Freeman.

Dement, W. C. (1983). Signs and symptoms of sleep disorders. In J. K. Walsh, A. D. Bertelson, & P. K. Schweitzer (Eds.), *Clinical aspects of sleep disorders: Proceedings of a symposium* (pp. 13–32). St. Louis, MO: Deaconess Hospital.

Dement, W. C., & Kleitman, N. (1957). Cyclic variations in EEG during sleep and their relation to eye movements, body motility, and dreaming. *Electroencephalography and Clinical Neurophysiology, 9*, 673–690.

Derogotis, L. R. et al. (1979). A survey of psychotropic drug prescriptions in an oncology population. *Cancer, 44*, 1919–1929.

Dye, C. J. (1978). Psychologists' role in the provision of mental health care for the elderly. *Professional Psychology, 5*, 38–49.

Edelstein, B. A., Keaton-Brasted, C., & Burg, M. M. (1984). Effects of caffeine withdrawal on nocturnal enuresis, insomnia, and behavior restraints. *Journal of Consulting and Clinical Psychology, 52*, 857–862.

Espie, C. A., & Lindsay, W. R. (1985). Paradoxical intention in the treatment of chronic insomnia: Six case studies illustrating variability in therapeutic response. *Behaviour Research and Therapy, 23*, 703–709.

Frankel, B. L., Coursey, R. D., Buchbinder, R., & Snyder, F. (1976). Recorded and reported sleep in chronic primary insomnia. *Archives of General Psychiatry, 33*, 615–623.

Franklin, J. (1981). The measurement of sleep onset latency in insomnia. *Behaviour Research and Therapy, 19*, 547–549.

Freedman, R., & Papsdorf, J. D. (1976). Biofeedback and progressive relaxation treatment of sleep-onset insomnia: A controlled all-night investigation. *Biofeedback and Self-Regulation, 1*, 253–271.

Gallup Organization. (1979). *Study of sleep habits.* Princeton, NJ: Author.

Gross, R. T., & Borkovec, T. D. (1982). Effects of a cognitive intrusion manipulation on the sleep-onset latency of good sleepers. *Behavior Therapy, 13*, 112–116.

Hauri, P. (1979). What can insomniacs teach us about the functions of sleep? In R. Drucker-Colin, M. Shkurovick, & M. B. Sterman (Eds.), *The functions of sleep* (pp. 251–271). New York: Academic Press.

Hauri, P. (1981). Treating psychophysiologic insomnia with biofeedback. *Archives of General Psychiatry, 38*, 752–758.

Hauri, P. (1982). *The sleep disorders.* Kalamazoo, MI: Upjohn.

Hauri, P., & Olmstead, E. (1980). Childhood-onset insomnia. *Sleep, 3*, 59–65.

Hauri, P., & Olmstead, E. (1983). What is the moment of sleep onset for insomniacs? *Sleep, 6*, 10–15.

Haynes, S. N., Adams, A. E., West, S., Kamens, L., & Safranek, R. (1982). The stimulus control paradigm in sleep-onset insomnia: A multimethod assessment. *Journal of Psychosomatic Research, 26*, 333–339.

Healey, E. S., Kales, A., Monroe, L. J., Bixler, E. O., Chamberlin, K., & Soldatos, C. R. (1981). Onset of insomnia: Role of life-stress events. *Psychosomatic Medicine, 43*, 430–451.

Hoelscher, T. J., & Edinger, J. D. (1986, March). Behavioral treatment of sleep-maintenance insomnia in the elderly. Paper presented at the annual meeting of the Society of Behavioral Medicine, San Francisco.

Horne, J. A., & Porter, J. M. (1976). Time of day effects with standardized exercise upon subsequent sleep. *Electroencephalography and Clinical Neurophysiology, 40*, 178–184.

Institute of Medicine. (1979). *Sleeping pills, insomnia, and medical practice.* Washington DC: National Academy of Sciences.

Jacobson, E. (1938). *Progressive relaxation*. Chicago: University of Chicago Press.

Jacobson, N. S., Follette, W. C., & Revenstorf, D. (1984a). Psychotherapy outcome research: Methods for reporting variability and evaluating clinical significance. *Behavior Therapy, 15,* 336–352.

Jacobson, N. S., Follette, W. C., Revenstorf, D., Baucom, D. H., Hahlweg, K., & Margolin, G. (1984b). Variability in outcome and clinical significance of behavioral marital therapy: A reanalysis of outcome data. *Journal of Consulting and Clinical Psychology, 52,* 497–504.

Johnson, L. C., & MacLeod, W. L. (1973). Sleep and awake behavior during gradual sleep reduction. *Perceptual and Motor Skills, 36,* 87–97.

Johnson, L. C., & Spinweber, C. L. (1983). Quality of sleep and performance in the Navy: A longitudinal study of good and poor sleepers. In C. Guilleminault & E. Lugaresi (Eds.), *Sleep/wake disorders: Natural history, epidemiology, and long-term evolution* (pp. 13–28). New York: Raven.

Kales, A., & Kales, J. D. (1974). Sleep disorders: Recent findings in the diagnosis and treatment of disturbed sleep. *New England Journal of Medicine, 290,* 487–499.

Kales, J. D., Kales, A., Bixler, E. O., Soldatos, C. R., Cadieux, R. J., Kashurba, G. J., & Vela-Bueno, A. (1984). Biopsychobehavioral correlates of insomnia, V: Clinical characteristics and behavioral correlates. *American Journal of Psychiatry, 141,* 1371–1376.

Kanner, A. D., Coyne, J. C., Schaefer, C., & Lazarus, R. S. (1981). Comparison of two modes of stress measurement: Daily hassles and uplifts versus major life events. *Journal of Behavioral Medicine, 444,* 1–39.

Karacan, I., Thornby, J. I., Anch, A. M., Booth, G. H., Williams, R. L., & Salis, P. J. (1976a). Dose-related sleep disturbances induced by coffee and caffeine. *Clinical Pharmacology and Therapeutics, 20,* 682–689.

Karacan, I., Thornby, J. I., Anch, A. M., Holzer, C. E., Warheit, G. J., Schwab, J. J., & Williams, R. L. (1976b). Prevalence of sleep disturbance in a primarily urban Florida county. *Social Science and Medicine, 10,* 239–244.

Kelley, J. E., & Lichstein, K. L. (1980). A sleep assessment device. *Behavioral Assessment, 2,* 135–146.

Killen, J. D., & Coates, T. J. (1979). The complaint of insomnia: What is it and how do we treat it? *Clinical Behavior Therapy Reviews, 1,* 1–15.

Kirmil-Gray, K., Coates, T. J., Thoresen, C. E., & Rosekind, M. R. (1978). Treating insomnia in adolescents. *Sleep Research, 7,* 237.

Kirmil-Gray, K., Eagleston, J. R., Thoresen, C. E., & Zarcone, V. P. (1985). Brief consultation and stress management treatments for drug-dependent insomnia: Effects on sleep quality, self-efficacy, and daytime stress. *Journal of Behavioral Medicine, 8,* 79–99.

Kripke, D. F. (1983). Why we need a tax on sleeping pills. *Southern Medical Journal, 76,* 632–636.

Kripke, D. F., Ancoli-Israel, S., Mason, W., & Messin, S. (1983). Sleep related mortality and morbidity in the aged. In M. H. Chase & E. D. Weitzman (Eds.), *Sleep disorders: Basic and clinical research* (pp. 415–429). New York: Spectrum.

Lacks, P. (in press). Daily sleep diary. In M. Hersen & A. S. Bellack (Eds.), *Dictionary of behavioral assessment techniques*. New York: Pergamon.

Lacks, P., Bertelson, A. D., Gans, L., & Kunkel, J. (1983). The effectiveness of three behavioral treatments for different degrees of sleep onset insomnia. *Behavior Therapy, 14,* 593–605.

Lacks, P., Bertelson, A. D., Sugerman, J. L., & Kunkel, J. (1983). The treatment of sleep maintenance insomnia with stimulus control techniques. *Behaviour Research and Therapy, 21,* 291–295.

Lacks, P., & Powlishta, K. (1986). *Improvement following behavioral treatment for insomnia: Clinical significance and long-term maintenance.* Manuscript submitted for publication.

Lacks, P., & Rotert, M. (1986). Knowledge and practice of sleep hygiene techniques in insomniacs and good sleepers. *Behaviour Research and Therapy, 24,* 365–368.

Largo, R. H., & Hunziker, U. A. (1984). A developmental approach to the management of children with sleep disturbances in the first three years of life. *European Journal of Pediatrics, 142,* 170–173.

Larsen, D., Attkisson, C., Hargreaves, W., & Nguyen, T. (1979). Assessment of client/patient satisfaction: Development of a general scale. *Evaluation and Program Planning, 2,* 197–207.

Lawton, M. P. (1972). Assessing the competence of older people. In D. Kent, R. Kastenbaum, & S. Sherwood (Eds.), *Research, planning and action for the elderly.* New York: Behavioral Publications.

Levin, D., Bertelson, A. D., & Lacks, P. (1984). MMPI differences among mild and severe insomniacs and good sleepers. *Journal of Personality Assessment, 48,* 126–129.

Lichstein, K. L., & Fischer, S. M. (1985). Insomnia. In M. Hersen & A. S. Bellack (Eds.), *Handbook of clinical behavior therapy with adults* (pp. 319–352). New York: Plenum.

Lichstein, K. L., Nickel, R., Hoelscher, T. J., & Kelley, J. E. (1982). Clinical validation of a sleep assessment device. *Behaviour Research and Therapy, 20,* 292–297.

Lichstein, K. L., & Rosenthal, T. L. (1980). Insomniacs' perceptions of cognitive versus somatic determinants of sleep disturbance. *Journal of Abnormal Psychology, 89,* 105–107.

Lichstein, K. L., & Sallis, J. F. (1982). Ocular relaxation to induce eye movements. *Cognitive Therapy and Research, 6,* 113–118.

Mahoney, M. (1977). Personal science: A cognitive learning therapy. In A. Ellis & R. Grieger (Eds.), *Handbook of rational-emotive therapy.* New York: Springer.

Marchini, E., Coates, T. J., Magistad, J. G., & Waldum, S. J. (1983). What do insomniacs do, think, and feel during the day? A preliminary study. *Sleep, 6,* 147–155.

Maxmen, J. (1981). *A good night's sleep.* Chicago: Contemporary Books.

Mellinger, G. D., Balter, M. B., & Uhlenhuth, E. H. (1985). Insomnia and its treatment: Prevalence and correlates. *Archives of General Psychiatry, 42,* 225–232.

Merritt, R. E., & Walley, D. D. (1977). *The group leader's handbook.* Champaign, IL: Research Press.

Miles, L. E., & Dement, W. C. (1980). Sleep and aging. *Sleep, 3,* 119–220.

Mintz, J., Steuer, J., & Jarvik, L. (1981). Psychotherapy with depressed elderly patients: Research considerations. *Journal of Consulting and Clinical Psychology, 49,* 542–548.

Mitchell, K. R. (1979). Behavioral treatment of presleep tension and intrusive cognitions in patients with severe predormital insomnia. *Journal of Behavioral Medicine, 2,* 57–69.

Monroe, L. J. (1967). Psychological and physiological differences between good and poor sleepers. *Journal of Abnormal Psychology, 72,* 255–264.

Monroe, L. J. (1969). Transient changes in EEG sleep patterns of married good sleepers: The effects of altering sleeping arrangement. *Psychophysiology, 6,* 330–337.

Morin, C. M., & Azrin, N. H. (1987). Stimulus control and imagery training in treating sleep-maintenance insomnia. *Journal of Consulting and Clinical Psychology, 55,* 260–262.

Morin, C. M., Duffee, S., Zande, M., & Azrin, N. H. (1986, November). Behavioral and cognitive treatments of geriatric insomnia. Paper presented at the annual meeting of the Association for the Advancement of Behavior Therapy, Chicago.

Nicassio, P. M., & Buchanan, D. C. (1981). Clinical application of behavior therapy for insomnia. *Comprehensive Psychiatry, 22,* 263–271.

Nicassio, P. M., Mendlowitz, D. R., Fussell, J. J., & Petras, L. (1985). The phenomenology of the pre-sleep state: The development of the Pre-Sleep Arousal Scale. *Behaviour Research and Therapy, 23,* 263–271.

O'Leary, A. (1985). Self-efficacy and health. *Behaviour Research and Therapy, 23,* 437–451.

Physician's desk reference. (1986). Oradell, NJ: Medical Economics Company.

Pillard, R. C., Atkinson, K. W., & Fisher, S. (1967). The effect of different preparations on film-induced anxiety. *Psychological Record, 17,* 35–41.

Price, V. A., Coates, T. J. Thoresen, C. E., & Grinstead, O. (1978). The prevalence and correlates of poor sleep among adolescents. *American Journal of Diseases of Children, 132,* 583–586.

Puder, R. (1984). *Overcoming ageism in psychotherapeutic practice: Some proposed guidelines for psychotherapy.* Unpublished manuscript, Washington University, St. Louis, MO.

Puder, R., Lacks, P., Bertelson, A. D., & Storandt, M. (1983). Short-term stimulus control treatment of insomnia in older adults. *Behavior Therapy, 14,* 424–429.

Rechtschaffen, A., & Kales, A. (Eds.). (1968). *A manual of standardized terminology, techniques and scoring system for sleep stages of human subjects.* Bethesda, MD: National Institute of Health.

Regestein, Q. R. (1980). Sleep and insomnia in the elderly. *Journal of Geriatric Psychiatry, 13,* 153–171.

Scharf, M. B., & Brown, L. (1986). Hypnotic drugs: Use and abuse. *Clinical Psychology Review, 6,* 39–50.

Schoicket, S. L., Bertelson, A. D., & Lacks, P. (1987). Is sleep hygiene a sufficient treatment for sleep maintenance insomnia? Manuscript submitted for publication.

Schultz, J. H., & Luthe, W. (1959). *Autogenic training: A psychophysiologic approach in psychotherapy.* New York: Grune & Stratton.

Shaffer, J. I., Dickel, M. J., Marik, N., & Slak, S. (1985). The effect of excessive motivation to fall asleep on sleep-onset. *Sleep Research, 14,* 102.

Soldatos, C. R., Kales, J. D., Scharf, M. B., Bixler, E. O., & Kales, A. (1980). Cigarette smoking associated with sleep difficulty. *Science, 207,* 551–552.

Spielberger, C. D., Gorsuch, R. L., & Lushene, R. E. (1970). *State-trait anxiety inventory-manual.* Palo Alto, CA: Consulting Psychologists Press.

Stam, H. J., & Bultz, B. D. (1986). The treatment of severe insomnia in a cancer patient. *Journal of Behavior Therapy and Experimental Psychiatry, 17,* 33–37.

Sugerman, J. L., Stern, J. A., & Walsh, J. K. (1985). Daytime alertness in subjective and objective insomnia: Some preliminary findings. *Biological Psychiatry, 20,* 741–750.

Teri, L., & Lewinsohn, P. M. (1986). Individual and group treatment of unipolar depression: Comparison of treatment outcome and identification of predictors of successful treatment outcome. *Behavior Therapy, 17,* 215–228.

Thoresen, C. E., Coates, T. J., Kirmil-Gray, K., & Rosekind, M. (1981). Behavioral self-management in treating sleep-maintenance insomnia. *Journal of Behavioral Medicine, 4,* 41–52.

Turk, D. C., Meichenbaum, D. L., & Genest, M. (1983). *Pain and behavioral medicine: A cognitive-behavioral perspective.* New York: Guilford.

Turner, R. M. & Ascher, L. M. (1979). Controlled comparison of progressive relaxation, stimulus control, and paradoxical intention therapies for insomnia. *Journal of Consulting and Clinical Psychology, 47,* 500–508.

Turner, R. M., DiTomasso, R. A., & Giles, T. (1982). Failures in the treatment of insomnia: A plea for differential diagnosis. In E. B. Foa (Ed.), *Failures in behavior therapy* (pp. 284–304). New York: Wiley.

Turner, R. M., DiTomasso, R., & Giles, T. (1982). Failures in the treatment of insomnia: A plea for differential diagnosis. In E. B. Foa (Ed.), *Failures in behavior therapy* (pp. 284–304). New York: Wiley.

VanOot, P. H., Lane, T. W., & Borkovec, T. D. (1984). Sleep disturbances. In P. Sutker & H. Adams (Eds.), *Handbook of psychopathology* (pp. 683–723). New York: Plenum.

Wallston, K. A., Wallston, B. S., & DeVellis, R. (1978). Development of the Multidimensional Health Locus of Control scales. *Health Education Monographs, 6,* 160–170.

Walsh, J. K. (1983). Overview of polysomnography and sleep physiology. In J. K. Walsh, A. D. Bertelson, & P. K. Schweitzer (Eds.), *Clinical aspects of sleep disorders: Proceedings of a symposium* (pp. 1–11). St. Louis: Deaconess Hospital.

Walsh, J. K., Sugerman, J. L., & Chambers, G. W. (1986). Evaluation of insomnia. *American Family Physician, 33,* 185–194.

Webb, W. B., & Agnew, H. W. (1975). Are we chronically sleep deprived? *Bulletin of the Psychonomic Society, 6,* 47–48.

Weil, G., & Goldfried, M. R. (1973). Treatment of insomnia in an eleven-year-old child through self-relaxation. *Behavior Therapy, 4,* 282–294.

Williams, B. R. (1986). Drugs and the elderly. *The Clinical Psychologist, 39*(4), 100–102.

Williams, R. L. (1978). Sleep disturbances in various medical and surgical conditions. In R. L. Williams and I. Karacan (Eds.), *Sleep disorders: Diagnosis and treatment* (pp. 285–301). New York: Wiley.

Wolfson, A. (1987). *The effects of parent training on the development of infant sleep patterns.* Unpublished doctoral dissertation, Washington University, St. Louis, MO.

Woolfolk, R. L., & McNulty, T. F. (1983). Relaxation treatment for insomnia: A component analysis. *Journal of Consulting and Clinical Psychology, 51,* 495–503.

Youkilis, H. D., & Bootzin, R. R. (1981). A psychophysiological perspective on the etiology and treatment of insomnia. In S. Haynes & L. Gannon (Eds.), *Psychosomatic disorders: A psychophysiological approach to etiology and treatment* (pp. 179–221). New York: Praeger.

Zwart, C. A., & Lisman, S. A. (1979). Analysis of stimulus control treatment of sleep-onset insomnia. *Journal of Consulting and Clinical Psychology, 47,* 113–118.

Author Index

153

Subject Index

About the Author

Patricia Lacks received her PhD in clinical psychology in 1966 from Washington University in St. Louis. She is currently a faculty member in the Department of Psychology at Washington University and is in part-time private practice as a clinical psychologist. Her chief interests are psychological assessment, health promotion, and behavioral treatment of depression, insomnia, and obesity. Dr. Lacks has been active in insomnia research since 1980 and has published and delivered a number of papers on these findings. In addition to many papers published on assessment and treatment outcome, Dr. Lacks is the author of the 1984 book *Bender Gestalt Screening for Brain Dysfunction*, as well as a widely used brochure *A Guide to Psychotherapy*.

Psychology Practitioner Guidebooks

Editors
Arnold P. Goldstein, Syracuse University
Leonard Krasner, Stanford University & SUNY at Stony Brook
Sol L. Garfield, Washington University in St. Louis

Cynthia D. Belar, William W. Deardorff & Karen E. Kelly — THE PRACTICE OF
CLINICAL HEALTH PSYCHOLOGY
Paul Karoly & Mark P. Jensen — MULTIMETHOD ASSESSMENT OF CHRONIC PAIN
William L. Golden, E. Thomas Dowd & Fred Friedberg — HYPNOTHERAPY: A
Modern Approach
Patricia Lacks — BEHAVIORAL TREATMENT FOR PERSISTENT INSOMNIA
Arnold P. Goldstein & Harold Keller — AGGRESSIVE BEHAVIOR: Assessment and
Intervention
C. Eugene Walker, Barbara L. Bonner & Keith L. Kaufman — THE PHYSICALLY AND
SEXUALLY ABUSED CHILD: Evaluation and Treatment
Robert E. Becker, Richard G. Heimberg & Alan S. Bellack — SOCIAL SKILLS
TRAINING TREATMENT FOR DEPRESSION